Imagination Becomes Reality

The Teaching of Master T'ung–tsai Liang

To: Burkey

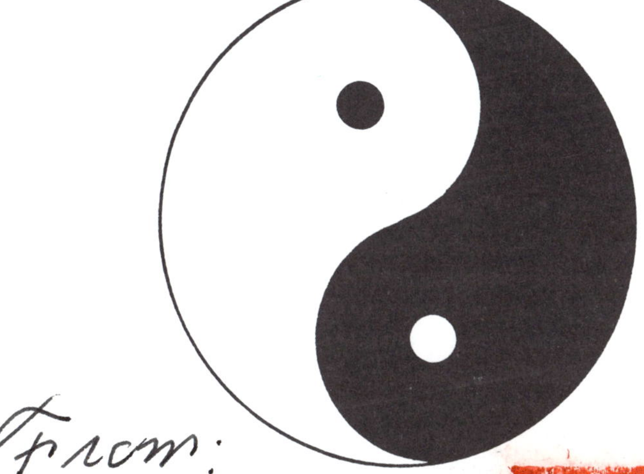

From:

Tungtsai Liang

Compiled By
Stuart Alve Olson

Edited By
Gerald Kuehl

T'AI CHI CH'UAN
THE TEACHINGS OF MASTER T.T. LIANG

IMAGINATION BECOMES REALITY

(150 Posture Solo Dance)

太極拳

COMPILED BY
STUART ALVE OLSON

EDITED BY
GERALD KUEHL

INTRODUCTION BY JONATHAN RUSSELL
(Eldest Student of Master Liang)

Library of Congress
Catalog Card Number

ISBN 0-938045-01-6

First printing: April, 1986

Printed in Canada by
D. W. Friesen & Sons Ltd.
Altona, Manitoba R0G 0B0
Canada

Bubbling-Well Press, Co.
P.O. Box 961
St. Cloud, Minnesota 56302

Table of Contents

Foreword

Bubbling-Well Press was established by Stuart Olson and myself, with the main objective of promoting related areas of Chinese culture. Our primary interest is the art of T'ai Chi Ch'uan.

My first experience with T'ai Chi came after more than a decade of practice in the hard, external styles. I found the attitude to be of a similar nature, rigid, with little yielding. It had little obvious effect to begin with but through time it began to take a noticeable toll physically and especially mentally. I commend the hard stylists who are able to maintain a yielding attitude in life, having not lost the traditional values the martial arts are centered upon. I had a great deal of difficulty in doing this.

In my opinion, our main concern should be that of attaining optimum health. A tense body and mind are simply not conducive to good health. It is also not the best way to develop self-defense skills. Confrontations usually occur quickly and a relaxed body and mind can give a considerable edge, with or without many years of training.

During my first experience with T'ai Chi Ch'uan it became apparent that relaxation is the cornerstone of the art. As Master Liang has stated, "It is impossible to acquire the essence of this art with a hard and unyielding attitude." To study this fascinating art is rewarding enough but to have a teacher of Master Liang's calibre is to be fortunate, indeed.

I have been learning T'ai Chi, under Master Liang, for two years. Stuart has lived and studied with this remarkable man for twice this period. We are very proud to publish this first volume, of a series, on the teachings of a true master of the art.

I wish to give special thanks to Master Liang for his effort in reviewing this work to ensure its accuracy. If this book was of metal, it would be of sword-like quality for it has been passed through the flames many times.

From my own standpoint, this book has been both enjoyable and informative; I hope you will find it equally so.

Jerry Kuehl

Foreword

Nearly seven years ago I became fascinated with the art of T'ai Chi Ch'uan. At that time I had no conception that my life would become so deeply involved with it. At first it was a mere fascination of its mystical aspects and later it became not only a means of livelihood but a way of life. Between teaching, writing and practicing T'ai Chi, I have found much truth in Master T. T. Liang's words, "At first I took T'ai Chi as a hobby to improve my health, gradually I became addicted to it and could not get rid of it." The same has been true for me.

I no longer look to T'ai Chi for any mystical experiences or wisdom, rather, my approach is that of searching for the more practical and humanistic aspects of this art.

T'ai Chi aside from all the supernatural tales surrounding it, is really nothing more than a basis for becoming a centered and aware human being. In my opinion, man learns little about himself or the spiritual realms when he is constantly looking outside his or her "self". T'ai Chi, like Zen, is only concerned with the here and now. Of course certain abilities, which the unlearned grasp as mystical feats, are cultivated within T'ai Chi, but they are nothing more than natural, inherent skills existing in everyone. Because of our tension, fears and bad habits these skills remain hidden, potential rather than kinetic. T'ai Chi helps draw them out. By becoming centered not only in the body but mind, developing awareness and sensitivity and ingraining the principles of T'ai Chi into one's actions and thoughts, it is possible to understand the 'here and now' and experience the so-called mystical skills of T'ai Chi. It all boils down to one thing, becoming a better human being by striving to make use of one's full potential in the most efficient way possible. From this we can come to understand why T'ai Chi can encompass not only health, martial art, mental accomplishment, but immortality as well.

For over four years now I have lived and studied with the great T'ai Chi master, T. T. Liang, who is a living example of the efficaciousness of this profound and subtle art. His teaching is always practical, never mystical — indeed this is what most erroneously conceive as his mystical side. His simplicity is difficult to comprehend by those who live such complicated lives, who refuse to yield with life and who are always on the defensive. Master Liang is like a willow tree wherein the branches yield to everything, yet the trunk remains rooted and stable. Those of us who have been fortunate enough to study with him understand this about him more than anything else.

The title of this book **Imagination Becomes Reality**, is the underlying teaching of Master T. T. Liang. The entire premise for attaining the skills of T'ai Chi Ch'uan is inherent within one's imagination, or more simply, it is purely a matter of mind-intent rather than gross physical skills which utilize external muscular force only. As Master Liang often states, ''When practicing T'ai Chi you must presume an opponent is in front of you. Gradually through continued practice the intrinsic energy, the ch'i and the technique will come out spontaneously in time of emergency.'' If caught unawares by an attack you will automatically react, with no time to think of a trained response. Hence, he summarizes this in the statement ''imagination becomes reality.''

This book is also just one in a series of works which will be titled, **''Imagination Becomes Reality.''** This particular volume focuses on the 150 posture solo form created by Master Liang. Other volumes will deal with the two-person (san-shou and ta-lu) set, pushing-hands and T'ai Chi principles for internal development. The entire series will be an indepth guide into the art of T'ai Chi Ch'uan empty-hand styles. Other books such as, **The Wind Sweeps Away the Plum Blossoms** (published 1985 by Bubbling-Well Press), **The Immortal Guiding the Way** (forthcoming) and **Splitting Open Mt. Hua** (forthcoming) will cover the solo and two-man sets of the weapons pertaining to T'ai Chi Ch'uan. In its entirety this will be a complete, indepth study of the T'ai Chi system, which has never been produced by one publishing house in either English or Chinese. Hopefully, in the future Bubbling-Well Press will be able to work with other teachers of the major systems and present their work in a similar fashion.

In conclusion I would like to thank the following people for all their kind help, generosity and faith: foremostly to Master T. T. Liang for providing many of his old, original written materials from which this book is entirely based. I must thank him deeply for his trust and patience during the process of compiling this work. Many thanks to Jonathan Russell for the many valuable photos shown in Chapter Three and his introduction piece to this book, his friendship and generosity are deeply appreciated; Gerald Kuehl, for his many hours of editing and final shaping of the book; Sara Kuehl for her endless patience during the many retypings of the manuscript; Paul Abdella for the cover design; Vern Peterson and Patrick Ryan for transcribing a number of the interview tapes; Char Ryan for typing the first draft of the manuscript; Fred Marych for all his work sorting photographs and his review of the text; Donna Balaski for her constant encouragement and for providing me with much help so that I would have more time in which to work on this book; I am forever in her debt.

Winter of 1985
St. Cloud, Minnesota
Stuart Alve Olson

Introduction:

For over twelve years I studied T'ai Chi Ch'uan with Master Liang in Boston, Massachusetts. The T'ai Chi that I learned, however, was often different from the T'ai Chi one might normally think of. I learned what could be called perhaps, "T.T. T'ai Chi," in essence living according to T'ai Chi principles. Master Liang at first appears to be a very complicated man, yet his actions are extraordinarily simple, like T'ai Chi itself. His playful intimidation is more often than not, a test of one's internal development. His consummate skill in the art of T'ai Chi, I believe, is matched by his ability to teach a "lesson in life" at the most disconcerting times. The following is a story which will help illustrate this unique aspect of T. T. Liang more clearly.

When living is Boston, Master Liang decided that he would take an English composition course at the University of Harvard. I was to take him there for his first class. Before setting out I asked him if he knew what building he was supposed to go to. T.T. told me that it had a steeple on top. Anyone who has ever been to Harvard University has undoubtedly noticed the vast number of buildings with white steeples on them. Driving in my car we came upon a mall, a huge lawned area lined with buildings, with a wide sidewalk running down the center. Not being able to locate the right building from the street, T.T. instructed me to drive down the sidewalk in order to find the building and avoid the long walk. At first I refused but T.T. told me not to worry that he would take full responsibility if the Harvard police stopped us. He said they would understand that such an old man should not be allowed to walk such a long distance.

So there we were driving down the sidewalk of Harvard mall. Sure enough the Harvard police came racing towards us and pulled my car over. Just as this happened T.T. jumped from the car, stood back, pointed at me and in a accusatorial manner yelled, "Arrest that man! He's a crazy man and should be put in jail!" He then walked down the sidewalk to the street to catch a bus home, leaving me the task of dealing with the police. He laughed for days after about how startled, confused and afraid I was during the whole ordeal.

With Master Liang you never know when he may catch you with one of his playful intimidating pranks, which is just like his skill in pushing-hands practice; you can never tell when a push is coming either.

The reason for Liang's playful intimidation is not just to test one's patience or ability to yield, rather its significance goes to the very root of the internal aspect of T'ai Chi, "abiding by the tan-tien." The essence of any practice of the internal arts (nei kung) is centered on this abiding by the tan-tien. In fact one cannot acquire the skills of root (central equilibrium), neutralization, counter-attack, nourishing the three treasures (ching, ch'i and shen), interpretation of energy and sticky energy etc. without adhering to this rule. They all have their source through abiding by this tan-tien. So Liang's playful intimidation is no more than a test to see if one can keep the ch'i down by not overreacting to any situation — a kind of verbal push-hands. Those who study T'ai Chi Ch'uan hear and read repeatedly the words, ''sink your ch'i,'' ''learn how to lose,'' ''yield,'' ''non-resistance,'' and ''abide by the tan-tien.'' It is these principles that Liang constantly attacks and tests.

Abiding by the tan-tien can only be done through use of the ''imagination.'' To the novice, no tan-tien can be either observed or felt, therefore one must first imagine this and gradually it will become real after long, mindful practice.

During the years I studied and helped teach T'ai Chi with Master Liang, he would constantly admonish his students to use their imagination so that eventually it would become a reality. Over and over again I would hear him say things like:

''When you are a beginner you should pretend that you have the skill of a great master and your progress will be very rapid.''

''You should pretend that your body is floating in water so that you feel a slight pressure against your every movement.''

''You imagine that as you push, your energy is directed by the mind and follows your intent.''

''You imagine that your center of gravity falls below the floor and you become firmly rooted.''

''You imagine . . . imagine . . . imagine.''

T'ai Chi Ch'uan is truly a form of imagination. From working with Liang it becomes clear that 10% of T'ai Chi is what you can see (the external movements) and the other 90% is what you cannot see, that is, the internal realm, the area that can be stimulated by correctly guiding your imagination. Real progress comes not from learning more and more, new and beautiful forms, (although T.T. is always dangling a new form that we don't know yet in front of our eyes) but from working with the most difficult and intangible area — the imagination.

Not surprisingly it is also the most difficult aspect for students to comprehend and is the secret of T'ai Chi. It is a secret that protects itself from being discovered because it is so simple. Most students feel that they have to acquire new knowledge, new techniques, when the tool that will really help them progress is with them all the time — their imagination. If this can be mastered, the internal realm of T'ai Chi Ch'uan will follow.

In the case of Stuart Olson, who is the only student to live with Master Liang for such an extended period of time, he has truly learned how to make his imagination become a reality, not only with his T'ai Chi but with his dreams as well. Two years ago he described to me his idea for a publishing house, Bubbling-Well Press, and that he wished to make it become a reality. This sounded great to me but I thought to myself that it was, as Liang often says, ''a bounced check.'' To my amazement what was in Stuart's imagination really has become a reality. Now if some of the other ideas in his head also become real — watch out! I for one definitely want to witness the realities of his imagination.

Jonathan Russell
Senior Student
Winter, 1985

Biography of Master T'ung Tsai Liang

T'ung-Tsai Liang was born in Hobei province, China, in 1900. His father was a merchant and his mother a very devout lay Buddhist. After college, Liang joined the maritime customs service at age twenty-four and served as a high ranking official for over 30 years. After the beginning of World War II he was transferred to Taiwan where he retired.

Since his move to the United States in 1963, Liang estimates that he has taught well over 3,000 students T'ai Chi Ch'uan. He has taught in such places as China, Taiwan, England, New York, Boston and presently in St. Cloud, Minnesota.

He and his teacher, Professor Cheng Man-Ch'ing, were the first official demonstrators of T'ai Chi Ch'uan in America, doing so at the United Nations in New York. Liang was Professor Cheng's first and eldest disciple, with more than twenty years service as his student. This earned him the title of Ta Shih Hsiung (Chief Disciple). While in New York at the United Nations, Liang served as both Professor Cheng's interpreter and teaching assistant. Later on Liang taught on his own at the United Nations and many well known east coast colleges including Boston College, Harvard University, Amherst, Springfield, Tufts, and Cumbres.

Because of his many location changes while serving as a customs official, Liang was able to meet many martial arts masters and practitioners. He studied under 15 prominent masters in all. The most notable were: Professor Cheng, Yuan Tao, Li Shou-Chen, Hsiung Yang-Ho, Han Ching-Tang, and Chang Tsun-Feng. He studied such arts as: T'ai Chi Ch'uan, Hsing-I chuan, Pa Kua Chang, Tang Lang Ch'uan (praying mantis), Shaolin Ch'uan, Chin Na and many related weapons. Some of Liang's more notable classmates were William C. C. Chen and Benjamin Lo.

About four years ago Liang moved to St. Cloud, Minnesota to semi-retire from teaching. His present activities include teaching T'ai Chi, painting, calligraphy, and translating and writing commentary on the Tao Te Ching.

Liang actually began his study of T'ai Chi Ch'uan at age twelve, but did not practice seriously until an illness at age forty almost took his life. Suffering from both a liver infection and pneumonia, he was given only two months to live. In order to save his own life he undertook vigorous T'ai Chi Ch'uan practice. As he explains in his book, **T'ai Chi Ch'uan for Health and Self-Defense,** "At first I took up T'ai Chi Ch'uan as a hobby; gradually I became addicted to it; now I can no longer get rid of it. I must keep on practicing for my whole life — it is the only way to preserve health.''

Within two years Liang's health had greatly improved. Now at age eighty-six he is a living example of the benefits of serious T'ai Chi Ch'uan practice. Even after 45 years of daily practice, his enthusiasm for the art is still strong.

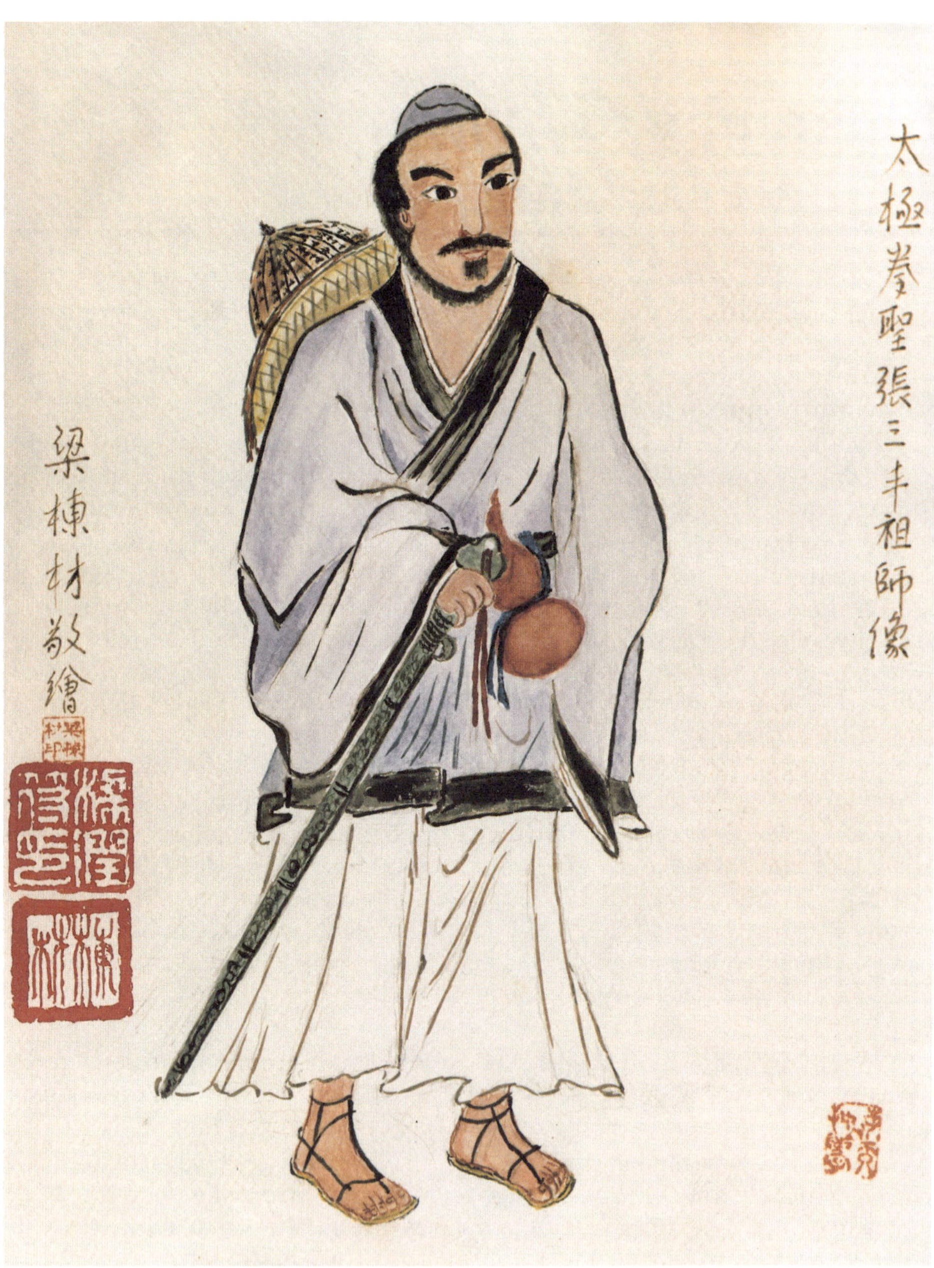

Chapter One

Interviews with Master T. T. Liang

What is T'ai Chi Ch'uan and how was it created?

First of all, T'ai Chi Ch'uan is commonly called just "T'ai Chi." It is an ancient form of classical dance created about seven hundred years ago by Chang San-feng, a Taoist priest of the Sung dynasty.

I will tell you how Chang San-feng created the circular version of T'ai Chi Ch'uan. Chang was a Taoist who travelled to many places by himself. He eventually arrived on Wu-Tang Mountain, in Hupei province, to study the old T'ai Chi classics and the original thirteen postures of T'ai Chi Ch'uan as practiced by the Taoists living there.

One day, while on Wu-Tang Mountain, he was reading the classics and heard a noise outside his hut. He looked outside and saw a magpie fighting with a snake on the ground. The bird would fly down from the tree and attempt to bite the snake. The snake could do little but by only moving his head, he could neutralize and avoid the attacks. He simply yielded, turning from side to side, to avoid the biting of the bird. After a little while, the bird flew back up into the tree, being too tired perhaps. Later on the bird again flew down to attack the snake. This time the bird tried using its wings to strike the snake. The snake again yielded, by turning from one side to another, neutralizing with his head as before. After many attempts, the bird could still not bite the snake. Both had become extremely tired, so they quit fighting and the bird flew away. From this incident, Chang San-feng began to comprehend, that is, he began to see the method of T'ai Chi. He adopted the hard and soft, combining them according to the T'ai Chi principles of the original thirteen postures and variations of yin and yang energy. He created what we now know as T'ai Chi Ch'uan, the round form. This is why it is called "meditation in action and action in meditation."

How did T'ai Chi Ch'uan get handed down from Chang San-feng to the present day?

Chang San-feng handed down his art to his disciple, Wang Chung-yueh. Wang wrote additional classics to preserve the art. This helped promote T'ai Chi because, now, in present times we have something to base our practice upon. Gradually the art moved to the Chen family, who hid it from outsiders for over three hundred years. After several generations it came to the Yang family. Now we may talk about the Yang family and Yang Lu-chan, the founder of the Yang style of T'ai Chi.

Yang Lu-chan was born in Hobei province. When he was still a young man, he travelled to Honan province. This occurred over one hundred years ago. The Chen family lived in Honan province and Yang journeyed there to learn T'ai Chi from the head of the family, Chen Chang-hsing. Chen was very skilled in T'ai Chi and had a good reputation.

The Chen family, however, only taught their relatives and not outsiders at this time. Yang Lu-chan definitely wanted to learn T'ai Chi from Chen but he knew he would receive little instruction if he just asked to be taught. Yang was very clever and pretended to be deaf and dumb. When he arrived at the village, the Chen's felt sorry for him and gave him a job as a servant. Yang secretly watched Chen Chang-hsing teaching his students every day. Eventually Chen discovered Yang spying on him and realized that he was not deaf and dumb. Yang Lu-chan then told him the whole story and asked Chen to teach him his art. Chen agreed, showed him a little bit and liked that Yang caught on so quickly. From then on Chen Chang-hsing taught Yang Lu-chan everything he knew about T'ai Chi. After about two years Yang had acquired all of Chen's art. One day Chen Chang-hsing called together his immediate family and relatives. He told them that a student named Yang Lu-chan had learned his entire art. He said that he had wanted to hand down his art to his family but that they were not able to learn it. He said Yang Lu-chan had managed to learn the art and was now leaving.

After leaving the Chen family village, Yang Lu-chan went back to Peking to teach the royal family and make T'ai Chi available to the public. In the palace he taught the princes, princesses and priests. Through time he taught far and wide and his skill became well known. No one could defeat him and he became known as "Yang the Unbeatable." He was the best of all.

Yang Lu-chan had three sons. The eldest, named Yang Feng-hou, died young. The second son was Yang Pan-hou and the third was called Yang Chien-hou. These two sons did not learn their father's entire art. It is not that they weren't skillful for they were great T'ai Chi masters. Pan-hou practiced all of time. In fact that is all he did was practice, his whole life through. Chien-hou reached the stage where if he stretched out his hand, he would hurt you, so few dared to learn from him.

Yang Chien-hou also had three sons, of which the second died young. Both Yang Shao-hou and Yang Cheng-fu, like their grandfather and father, practiced T'ai Chi and mastered the art. There are many stories of combat concerning these two sons because they liked to fight. Yang Cheng-fu, when young, didn't like to practice T'ai Chi and didn't really learn it from his father until he was older. It wasn't until his father had died that Yang Cheng-fu regretted not having had the art handed down to him. He wished to hand it down to his children. To make up for this loss, Yang Cheng-fu practiced very hard every day and learned as much as he could from the other family members. Eventually he became an expert. Afterwards Cheng-fu changed the style to be even softer than that of his grandfather and father. His form looked soft but internally it was very hard. That is why it was often said that his arms felt like iron bars wrapped in cotton. He was very kind and his temper very mild, so many students came to learn from him.

Yang Cheng-fu had four sons. The eldest was named Chen-ming; the second, Chen-chi; the third son was called Chen-to and the fourth, Chen-kou.

From this lineage the Yang style of T'ai Chi has progressed and remained popular. Of course the best one was the grandfather, Yang Lu-chan. He handed down his art to his sons but they never reached his level of skill. The last generation, now living in Hong Kong, have gradually made the style more and more popular, even in the United States. In my opinion the Yang style, of T'ai Chi Ch'uan is the best.

Why should we practice T'ai Chi Ch'uan and what are the processes for learning?

The fundamental principles for learning T'ai Chi fall into four categories: health, self-defense, mental accomplishment and immortality.

First, we must discuss health. In the T'ai Chi classics it says, "When the lowest vertebrae are plumb erect, the spirit of vitality reaches the top of the head." When the top of the head feels as if it is suspended from above, the whole body will be light and nimble. This is the way to strengthen the spine and by doing this, one not only strengthens the internal organs but the brain itself. The T'ai Chi classics also state that the "ch'i must be stimulated." The ch'i is an inherent oxygen in the body necessary for stamina and vitality. The stimulation of the ch'i can be compared to the action of wind on the smooth surface of a lake. As the wind moves across the water, it creates waves, blowing them upward and downward in a systematic order of troughs and crests. The ch'i, latent in the body, is not sufficiently forceful in itself to increase the flow of blood but if persistently stimulated it can produce heat. This can be very effective in circulating the blood evenly throughout the entire body. The same principle is illustrated by the conversion of water into steam. The invisible power latent in water is made active enough to drive the piston of a powerful engine.

To practice T'ai Chi Ch'uan, it is best to rise early and practice outdoors. To do this it is necessary to keep away from the alcoholic, drug addict and gambler. One must get rid of bad habits. Assimilate the new and let go of the old.

I introduced the system of using beats so that the postures could be practiced slowly to music. By doing the exercises effortlessly and evenly coordination is created between the mind and the body. "Early to bed, early to rise, along with a round of T'ai Chi morning and evening, makes a man or woman, healthy, wealthy and wise!" This is for health.

After one has acquired good health, one may seek the self-defense aspects. By practicing the one hundred and fifty postures of T'ai Chi one will develop central equilibrium, that is a firm rooting of the feet. From pushing-hands, yielding and neutralizing attacks will be learned. Practicing the one hundred and seventy-eight posture two-person dance is also necessary. This will develop intrinsic energy in the sinews and tendons because one will learn to use the whole body as one unit. A strike with only the hand will make the body become tense. This is not only ineffective for functional use but harmful to one's health. Various energies will be developed over a period of time and this will aid in acquiring the self-defense aspect of the art.

The third stage is mental accomplishment. After attaining good health and acquiring the techniques of self-defense it is necessary to realize mental accomplishment. To accomplish T'ai Chi physically and technically is relatively easy in comparison to attaining it mentally. From my more than forty years of experience, learning and practicing T'ai Chi, I have formulated ten theorems for my daily guiding principles to help me to know how to deal with people and myself. The principles are as follows:

1. No one can be perfect. Take what is good and discard what is bad.
2. If I believe entirely in books, it is better not to read books. If I rely entirely on teachers, it is better not to have teachers.
3. To remove a mountain is easy but to change a man's temperament is more difficult.
4. If there is anything wrong with me, I do not blame others, I only blame myself.
5. If I want to live longer I must learn T'ai Chi and accomplish it both physically and mentally. To accomplish it mentally is much more difficult.
6. I must learn how to yield, be tactful, not be aggressive, to lose (small loss, small gain, great loss, great gain) and how not to take advantage of others. I must also learn how to give for the more one gives the more one will have.
7. Life begins at seventy. Everything is beautiful! Health is a matter of utmost importance and all of the rest is secondary. Now I must find out how to enjoy excellent health in my whole life and discover the way to immortality.
8. Make one thousand friends but not one enemy.
9. One must practice what one preaches, otherwise, it is empty talk or a bounced check.
10. To conceal the faults of others and praise their good points is the best policy.

By learning and practicing T'ai Chi and by following the ten theorems as mentioned above, your hot temper will gradually become mild. Hatred, jealousy, anger and all depraved thoughts will disappear. Your evil temperament will be reformed, leaving evil to follow the good. Your mind will become upright and pure.

When you reach the age of seventy, you will enjoy a happy, peaceful and quiet life. At that age you will realize that fame, wealth, authority and honor are all dust. You will then purify your mind and lessen your desires so that you can fully enjoy your life and appreciate nature. That is why I say that life begins at seventy. The world is beautiful.

Now we come to the last stage, that of immortality. The ultimate goal for learning and practicing T'ai Chi is to become an immortal. Let me recount an old belief!

When Chang San-feng had sat in meditation on Wu-Tang Mountain for nine years, he still could not obtain his final goal, that of becoming an immortal. One day he got up from his meditation and began practicing the posture "Step Back To Chase The Monkey Away." After less than thirty minutes he suddenly felt that all of the joints in his body had widely opened. His spirit immediately took flight to another world, paradise and he became an immortal.

Ordinarily the two bones of the buttocks are pinched and the ch'i cannot sink downward. When Chang San-feng practiced this posture he put one foot behind, with the feet parallel and the toes pointing directly ahead. His stance was such that the distance between his two legs was of shoulder-width. This allowed the ch'i to sink downward to the legs and into the "bubbling-well" points on the soles of the feet, thereby pushing the blood throughout the entire body without hindrance. This is how Chang San-feng finally reached his goal and became an immortal.

The principles and theories of T'ai Chi are so profound and abstruse and the applications so subtle and ingenious that it is important to find the correct method of learning and practicing. If what is learned is not quite accurate and correct, then one's ability may be severely handicapped. The fundamental use of T'ai Chi will be lost and it will be useless to talk about mental accomplishment and the way to immortality.

Whether it is possible to achieve immortality, by learning and practicing T'ai Chi, is not the main concern. The greatest hope is that of reaching one hundred years of age or more. This is the highest level of longevity.

Nevertheless, a person's life and death are predetermined. Wealth, poverty, fame and honor are in the hands of heaven. I strongly believe in cause and effect. We must live virtuously, enjoy life, appreciate nature and wait for our final allotment so that we have not spent the best days of our life in vain.

What do you mean by cause and effect?

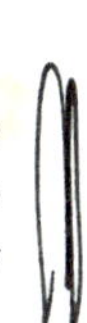

When you do something, good or bad, it will in turn come back to you. This means that you will get a result or an effect. Doing good things or acts of virtue produce good results. I believe strongly in this. Be good, learn to yield and enjoy life without being bad to others. That is all.

How would you know a true T'ai Chi master?

The arms of a true T'ai Chi master are like iron bars wrapped in cotton. They are extremely flexible but internally strong and heavy. When grasping an opponent's hand as in pushing-hands practice, the T'ai Chi master's hands are very light but the opponent cannot get away from him. He can release intrinsic energy from his spine like the bullet from the muzzle of a gun. His strike is lightning swift and clear cut like the breaking of a stick, without the slightest exertion of muscular force.

As soon as an opponent feels a slight stir of his body, he is already pushed more than ten feet away without feeling any pain. When the T'ai Chi master attaches his hands lightly to the hands of an opponent, without grasping them, they are as firm as glue. It is impossible to remove them and they will cause a terrible aching and numbness in the opponent's arms. Trying to subdue and restrain a T'ai Chi master is like attempting to catch the wind. You end up with nothing at all. It is like stepping on a gourd in the water; it is so slippery that it is impossible to get a firm hold or footing. This is the real meaning of self-defense concerning T'ai Chi. These are the words of my teacher's teacher, Yang Cheng-fu. They are accurate and precise. My teacher proved them true, gaining my great respect.

Would you list the complete set of T'ai Chi Ch'uan?

If you wish to study T'ai Chi for health and self-defense it is necessary to learn the entire set of T'ai Chi Ch'uan. The complete set is as follows:

1. T'ai Chi solo dance (right and left styles with 150 postures in each style).
2. Pushing-Hands (active steps in fixed position, 8 movements).
3. Ta Lu (3 sets, total of 26 postures).

4. T'ai Chi Two-Person Dance (178 postures).
5. T'ai Chi Double-Edged Sword Dance (right and left styles, 60 postures in each).
6. T'ai Chi Sword Fencing (46 postures).
7. T'ai Chi Knife Dance (right and left styles, 32 postures in each).
8. T'ai Chi Knife Fencing (24 postures).
9. T'ai Chi Staff Solo Exercise (3 movements).
10. T'ai Chi Staff Fencing (8 postures).

All of these exercises can be practiced to music.

Why is it necessary to practice T'ai Chi with weapons?

To practice T'ai Chi without weapons, that is to practice only the empty-hand sets, is to strengthen the muscles of the body and not the sinews and tendons. Weapon practice will strengthen the sinews and tendons. When the body, hands and weapon act as one unit, the intrinsic energy will reach to the tip of the weapon. Therefore, intrinsic energy can be developed to the fullest extent and to the highest level. Practice without weapons will mean that the intrinsic energy will reach only as far as the finger tips.

For example, this sword, here in my hand, must be used with the whole body as one unit. It should not be used with only the arm. In ancient times people trained to be soft and delicate with the sword. They did not try merely to develop strength and generate force. Daily practice will enable the intrinsic energy to come out. If it is not developed, a person will be unable to push an opponent far away when engaged in empty-hand fighting. This is why it is necessary to practice T'ai Chi with weapons, so use the sword, sabre and staff.

Why did you take up T'ai Chi Ch'uan?

When I was a young man I practiced many hard styles like karate, judo and Chinese Shaolin kung-fu. I also played many sports such as soccer, basketball and tennis. I began working with the Chinese Maritime Customs in my early twenties. Eventually I reached the high position of Chief Tide Surveyor. During this time, I dissipated and drank too much and at the age of forty-five I became very sick. I was committed to a hospital for more than fifty days. During this time I nearly died. After recovering and leaving the hospital I was still weak to the point where I could no longer do the hard styles of kung-fu. I thought that the best way for me to regain my health would be to learn T'ai Chi Ch'uan. I did so and eventually learned from almost fifteen teachers. The best of them all, in my opinion, was Prof. Cheng Man-ch'ing. I have, to the most extent, adopted his method of performing the T'ai Chi Ch'uan exercise.

It took me ten years to regain my health. After that I continued to practice. Now I am over eighty-five years of age and enjoy perfect health. If not for T'ai Chi Ch'uan I can easily say that my life would have ended forty years ago. Of all of the forms of exercise I consider T'ai Chi Ch'uan the best. It saved my life and that is why I strongly advocate that everyone take up this exercise so that they may also enjoy good health.

What is it that you do in this exercise?

The essence of T'ai Chi is to relax, sink all of the weight downward and sink the ch'i into the tan t'ien. The whole body must be entirely relaxed. This is very beneficial for health.

What is the difference between T'ai Chi Ch'uan and other popular forms of exercises in terms of its advantages?

T'ai Chi is different from yoga and other forms of exercise. It is not only excellent for one's health but develops self-defense skills as well.

Yoga is good, without question and jogging is fine too. Most of the common forms of exercise, however, are beneficial only when the person is young. At an older age, exercises like jogging, can lose their health benefits. Jogging can be hard on the joints and place undue stress on the heart.

T'ai Chi, however, is beneficial, no matter what age it is practiced. Whether young, old, male or female, it is an exercise that promotes good health. Also, practice after a period of time will develop self-defense skills. Jogging and yoga will not teach this.

How can these slow, dance-like movements be used for health?

That is an interesting question. Slow motion is good for health because first of all by practicing slowly the ch'i can sink to the tan-tien. This energy, ch'i, will gradually penetrate into the sinews and tendons making the bones very hard. Sinking the ch'i will also allow the blood to circulate freely throughout the entire body. This is very important for one's health.

T'ai Chi Ch'uan, as a martial art, emphasizes relaxation. If the body is tense, the ch'i will rise up impeding blood circulation. This is common with the hard styles like kung-fu and karate. These arts involve using external, muscular force, called "li" which is issued from the bone. By striking this way it is possible to hurt oneself and the resulting tension is not beneficial.

By utilizing slow movement in a relaxed manner, T'ai Chi Ch'uan is very good for one's health.

The yin and yang symbol represents T'ai Chi. Why is this so?

Yin and yang are in the T'ai Chi "Tu" with one half being yin and the other half being yang. Yang is the substantial and yin the insubstantial. Yang is hard and yin is soft. All of T'ai Chi is based on this yin and yang principle.

The principle relates to T'ai Chi Ch'uan with regards to it's roundness. T'ai Chi must have roundness in it's form. It must be practiced with circularity and yin and yang within.

The postures must be circular and not straight forward. This is especially true for the beginner. The circles should be large to begin with and gradually condensed into small ones. After one has acquired the art, the small circles become invisible.

Even the body has yin and yang aspects to it. When learning T'ai Chi one must realize the practical use of the postures. To learn this it is necessary to know the opponent, that is, where the yin and yang areas are on his body. A push will be effective if done on the yang part but you will not be able to push him over if you strike his yin area.

Yin and yang can be found throughout T'ai Chi with everything performed in circles so the T'ai Chi "Tu," well represents the art.

What does gaining a root mean?

A root means central equilibrium. When you stand and someone tries to push you over but can't, this is central equilibrium. Your feet will be rooted just like a tree. It is possible to acquire this by performing the T'ai Chi Ch'uan exercises daily at least two or three times. A root is very important and little else can be achieved in T'ai Chi until a person obtains one. When no one can push you over, you can learn how to yield. From yielding you will learn how to counter-attack. Everything is done step by step.

So, first, a beginner must acquire a root, through daily practice of T'ai Chi Ch'uan. Even though I'm over eighty-five years old, a young man cannot push me over because I've been practicing for so many years. I've naturally developed a root. If you don't believe me, try it.

What is the meaning of using the whole body as one unit? Is this related to intrinsic energy?

The T'ai Chi classic by Chang San-feng says, ''The entire body must be used as one unit.'' Therefore when you turn leftward, the body, waist and head must turn simultaneously. The head must remain in the same position as before the turn. When moving backwards or forwards, left or right, the body should move as one unit. In this way intrinsic energy will be developed. Intrinsic energy comes from the sinews and tendons. It originates from the feet, flows into the legs, then waist and is issued by the spine. The whole body must relax and push forward as one unit for intrinsic energy to be released.

To develop this you must learn that when you strike out to not use muscular energy. This force is from the bone and means that the hands are working independently of the rest of the body. The ch'i will rise up and the body will become tense. After a few strikes you will become tired.

If, however, you strike with intrinsic energy, the ch'i will sink into the tan-tien; it will go downward not upward. Striking in this manner is like using a whip. It is tremendously powerful.

When speaking of the martial aspects of T'ai Chi Ch'uan, you say that the substantial and insubstantial must be clearly differentiated. What do you mean by that?

Substantial means hard or solid and insubstantial means soft or empty. It is very important to realize this when engaged in pushing-hands. A large part of pushing-hands practice involves trying to find the opponent's center of gravity. As soon as his center is found, a push will be successful because he will not be able to neutralize it. If on the other hand, his body is found to be soft and empty, he will be able to neutralize your attack. Knowing his substantial and insubstantial, that is, where he is solid and where he is empty is necessary for an effective attack.

If you find the substantial, pushing will be easy but if not, it will be necessary to make him move by pulling his hands or by using some other tactic. This will aid in finding the substantial part of his body so he can be pushed over.

To ensure an attack's success, you must know your opponent. Remember, if you cannot test or interpret your opponent's yin and yang, substantial and insubstantial, you do not know him.

What is mind–intent?

When you practice T'ai Chi Ch'uan, on a solo basis, it should be done by what is called "imagination." This means that when you wish to push someone over, you do it with your mind. You do not actually use muscular force; you only use your mind. Through being completely relaxed, your mind will gradually presume that there is an opponent in front of you. You will push him over, even though there is no one there.

Let us suppose that I wish to push you over through use of my mind only. Even though I do not use energy I will push you for a great distance because the ch'i will follow immediately the mind's command. This stage can be reached only by consistent, daily practice without using the slightest bit of energy.

At this level, when you practice pushing–hands with someone, your mind will immediately take over; the ch'i will come out and you will knock him over instantly. This is imagination becoming reality.

Has T'ai Chi affected you personally?

T'ai Chi has affected me a great deal. When I was young I had a very bad temper which got me into a lot of trouble. I was always ready to fight and generally did a lot of notorious things. Even when I joined the Maritime Customs Service, with a good position and pay, I would get into a lot of trouble. Twice I was disrated, meaning my pay would not be increased. I didn't care. When I reached the highest position that I could, I thought of myself as a real authority. At this time I had bodyguards and when I gave an order, it had to be carried out immediately. I did not believe in anyone but myself. I became very sick during this time and was committed to a hospital. When I was released I took up T'ai Chi.

I have been learning and practicing T'ai Chi for more than forty years now. After the first five years I thought that I knew everything and started to criticize this man and that man as being unskilled. So actually in all this time my attitude hadn't really changed. I began to think that only I was any good. After another ten years of learning and practicing, I began to realize that I knew only a little about T'ai Chi and life in general. Instead of criticizing others, I started to criticize myself because I realized that I was not qualified to judge with my smattering of knowledge. Besides, I had no time to criticize others because I had to practice and painstakenly learn from teachers, books and the T'ai Chi classics. The more I learned, the less I felt that I knew.

The theory and philosophy of T'ai Chi are so profound and abstruse and the functional use so subtle and ingenious, that I felt I must continue studying and practicing T'ai Chi forever. I am still of that opinion. It is the only way to improve and better myself. So, yes, I can say that T'ai Chi has, indeed, affected me a great deal.

You stated earlier that T'ai Chi Ch'uan has a Taoist origin. What does the Taoist philosophy of Lao Tzu and T'ai Chi Ch'uan have in common?

Everything you do in T'ai Chi Ch'uan has an equivalent in the philosophy of Lao Tzu or simply Taoism in general. In my book, T'ai Chi Ch'uan for Health and Self Defense, I discuss the similarities between Lao Tzu's Taoism and the T'ai Chi classics in length. I will say, however, that the greatest similarity occurs at the highest stage of T'ai Chi practice, that of immortality. The final goal of both T'ai Chi and Taoism is immortality.

Chang San-feng, a Taoist, created T'ai Chi Ch'uan. He later became an immortal through his practice of T'ai Chi so it is said that T'ai Chi Ch'uan is a Taoist method for attaining immortality.

In this atomic age why should anyone practice T'ai Chi considering how life has changed since ancient China?

Today, everyone is too aggressive. No one wishes to yield. Everybody wishes to take advantage of others. This is common in all societies and all countries. If things continue the way they are going, there will be a third world war. This has been predicted as being inevitable. If this war occurs, it will be far worse than the last because of the development of nuclear warfare. The atomic bombs of today will not be like the two dropped on Japan in World War II. They had relatively little destructive ability. This time war will possibly demolish the world and many human beings will perish.

If everyone learned to relax, yield and lose, this predicted third world war would be avoided. If everyone learned not to be aggressive by following the principles of T'ai Chi Ch'uan, wars could be abolished. This is why I strongly advocate the practice of T'ai Chi.

Would you please explain the ideas of hearing energy, sticking energy, neutralizing energy and attacking energy?

Hearing energy involves feeling the opponent's energy. When someone touches you, you do not hear a sound but immediately you know him. This means that you are aware of his intent and actions. You will feel his slightest stir and, therefore, will be able to act. The development of this form of energy will mean being able to determine the real from the unreal, that is, whether the opponent is faking or not. It will enable you to know in what direction to neutralize by just how the opponent touches your body. You will know whether he is strong or weak.

Sticking energy means the opponent cannot get rid of you. It is as if you were plaster attached to his body. If you move, he must follow. If you go forward, he must retreat and if you retreat, he must come forward. With this type of energy, the opponent is under your complete control.

Neutralizing energy involves getting rid of your opponent's energy when it comes to you. Doing this disallows his energy from coming in contact with your body. This is acomplished by learning how to yield and lose.

Attacking energy means to use a counter-offensive technique on your opponent. You must use intrinsic energy which involves using the whole body as one unit. This is not easy because, first, it is necessary to master all of the techniques.

When you speak of attacking energy, you say that there are many different types of attacking energy, such as prolonged energy, abrupt energy, lowering energy and sinking energy. What do all of these mean?

These energies all depend on the action of your opponent. To prolong, means to take your opponent a long, long way. Sometimes it is necessary to use just a jerking movement which is very abrupt, letting go immediately afterwards. Depending upon your opponent, you may have to go further by either lowering, raising, sinking or pulling. If you encounter resistance you must use a technique; if there is no resistance, you can just push him over.

You say that when you push, there must be a circle and when you punch, the second you make contact the fist turns. Are these two actions related?

Yes, both employ corkscrew energy. If it is used properly it will penetrate directly into the opponent's body like a screw. You do not use just the hand in this strike, though. If you do, you will be using external muscular force which will not affect the opponent internally. You must use the intrinsic energy, that is, the whole body as one unit as I have mentioned before. Externally, nothing will be apparent but internally there will be an injury.

It is a tremendously powerful strike. Everytime you push or strike, you must use this circle or corkscrew motion. Even when pushing in a straight line, it is necessary to use this motion. The hand must turn slightly but with the whole body. By doing this, you will be utilizing the intrinsic energy to the greatest degree. This is rather difficult to express unless a teacher demonstrates it, however.

When you push someone, you do not appear to move much at all. How is it that you can push someone over like this?

When you actually push someone it is important that you do not lean forward or actually push forward. The push should be executed with just a turning motion, a release of the breath and a sinking motion. You must use your whole body as one unit, sink down and ''push'', without going forward.

It is important to keep your equilibrium during the push or you will put yourself into a defective position. Move as one unit, keep your back perfectly erect and the push will be performed correctly.

The power of the push originates from the foot moves to the leg and is issued by the spine. It has nothing to do with the hands. When I push, you will see little movement and sometimes none at all. It looks invisible but I will push you far away. My teacher taught me this and did it to me many times. I would not see his hands move but I would be pushed for a great distance. Practicing pushing-hands and the forms will gradually develop this energy. This can only be accomplished, however, through constant practice.

Why are these terms defined as energies? Why are they not called ''forces'' or something of that nature?

When you relax, you do not use force. Force comes from the bone and energy comes from the sinews and tendons. To generate energy one must not only be sensitive, relaxed and alert but use the whole body as one unit. Force involves tension and the use of external musculature. Energy is internal and is issued mostly from the spine.

Force is used in the external martial styles, like karate and kung-fu, because individual limbs are employed with limited use of the whole body. Internal systems, such as T'ai Chi Ch'uan, develop various energies through relaxation and the use of the entire body as one unit.

Master Liang can you describe pushing-hands?

The second goal of T'ai Chi Ch'uan is self-defense. For self-defense you must learn pushing-hands. This exercise consists usually of four movements. They are ward-off, rollback, press and push.

In practice they would be used as follows:

1. You would Push me and I would Roll-back.
2. Then, you would perform Press on me and I would neutralize it.
3. I would Push you and you would do Roll-back.
4. I would Press and you would neutralize.

These movements are repeated, back and forth in this manner. The reason for doing this exercise is to learn to neutralize, relax, yield and lose.

In pushing-hands you must entice the opponent into advancing and then, when his energy is emptied, adhere to him and issue energy. Adhere, join, stick and follow without letting go and without resistance. This is the correct method for pushing-hands.

The most important movement of the four, according to my teacher, is the roll-back posture. When you have mastered the roll-back posture and its application, you will have mastered one half of T'ai Chi.

This is how roll-back is used. When you push me and I can't take it anymore, without losing my balance, I neutralize with the roll-back technique. I must let your energy go to the side and not to my body. If the push comes on my left arm, I neutralize with my left palm turning upwards. This is a secret technique that came from the Yang family. This movement is very important if the posture is to be effective.

What do you mean by learning how to lose and how is this useful for self-defense?

Learning how to lose means to not use force against force. When energy comes to your body, do not resist. This is called ''small loss, small gain, big loss, big gain.''

When your opponent pushes, you must yield. Eventually no one will be able to put their energy on your body. Gradually your body will become soft and you will bend like a willow tree.

In the T'ai Chi classics it says, ''your waist will be as though boneless.'' To attain this degree of pliability, you must be very soft but once it has been attained, no one will be able to touch you. This is all accomplished by learning how to lose.

The classics also say, ''To yield means to attack; to withdraw means to attack.'' These two movements occur simultaneously. To yield, let your opponent come to you and then neutralize his energy; lead him into your trap, then go forward and attack him. In this way, losing will enable a small person to overcome a much larger opponent. If force against force is used, the stronger man will win.

What is the procedure for learning pushing-hands?

The process for learning pushing-hands involves three steps. The first step is to acquire a root or ''central equilibrium.'' This means that it is very difficult for your opponent to push you over. What is important is that when you practice pushing-hands you do not use this root. This would be force against force and in direct opposition of T'ai Chi principles.

The next step is to learn how to lose. As mentioned earlier, you will develop softness and suppleness in yielding to your opponent's push.

The third step is the counteroffense. This involves attacking and pushing your opponent over. It is not that easy, though. It means that you will have to discover your opponent's yin and yang areas or substantial and insubstantial aspects.

You must find his center of gravity. A successful push requires that you know this. Next, you must determine the line. Altogether, there are twenty-five lines. The line you choose will depend on the opponent's position so the push will not necessarily be straight.

Next, it is important to avoid being double-weighted. You must relax and use the whole body as one unit in your push. This will allow you to use intrinsic energy. When these conditions are met, you can push effectively.

This all means that in order to break your opponent's root, you must know your superior position and his defective one. These are things to know or be capable of doing in order to push successfully:

1. The substantial and insubstantial of the opponent's body.
2. Center of balance.
3. Lines of attack or opponent's defective position.
4. Use your whole body as one unit (intrinsic energy).

Your counterattack will be of little use if you do not pay attention to these points.

After a long period of training, as soon as your hand touches the opponent's body, you will know whether your push will be effective or not. Everything will be in your mind, already, so you will know instantly in what direction to push. If you do not know, it will be a matter of ''blind man's buff'', that is, you will only be guessing.

What is sticky energy?

Sticky energy is divided into three levels: lowest, middle and highest. The lowest level requires that one touch the opponent's body with the hand in order to push him over. There are two methods for this. One is borrowing his energy in order to issue your own energy. This is called the ''receive-attack'' technique. The other is to entice your opponent to issue his energy and, then, after neutralizing all his energy to one side, you knock him over with the ''roll-back'' technique. These two techniques are the most elemental methods used in T'ai Chi pushing-hands.

The middle level of sticky energy is described by the saying, ''as soon as one touches the clothing of the other man, he is already in your trap.'' No sooner does your palm attach to his clothing than he is uprooted. At this level he can be thrown in any of eighteen ways.

A person with the highest level of sticky energy can use his flat palm to lift anything without exerting strength through the fingers. One of the Yang family disciples, Chen Hsui-feng, relied only on the sticky energy of one palm to raise a heavy armchair and carry it from one spot to another. So, it is said in the T'ai Chi classics, ''with the mind-intent, the ch'i follows.'' His palm was full of electromagnetic-like energy to which the armchair was irresistibly attracted. This is the most developed form of sticky energy. It is an art that is almost completely lost.

Please explain a little about the two-person dance set.

The two-person dance involves moving with a partner. It may be performed to music. Every posture in the two-person set consists of three movements done in slow motion. They are: neutralize, seize and attack. The dance will teach that when someone strikes at you, it is necessary to first neutralize the attack, then seize (attach to) the limb or opponent's body and strike back. You will be able to do this properly only after a great deal of practice. Although it is done slowly in the two-person set, after a period of time, all three movements will be performed very quickly.

When it comes to learning the practical use of T'ai Chi, the two-person dance is excellent. I will give an example of its useage. When an opponent strikes with his hands, you must know the correct way to neutralize, that is, to neutralize your body in order to avoid his strike.

For the second movement, you must put your body into a superior position. This is done by adjusting your waist and legs. Immediately hold his arm or lightly touch his body in order to understand (interpret) his center of balance and substantial and insubstantial aspects.

The third movement involves putting your opponent into a defective position. Feel his joints and then immediately strike. When striking, remember what I have said before, that the body must be relaxed and used as one unit.

The T'ai Chi classics say, ''The hands and feet should be relaxed and the waist must act as one unit so that when advancing and retreating you will obtain a good opportunity and a superior position.'' If you fail to gain these advantages, your body will be in a state of disorder and confusion. The only way to correct this fault is by adjusting your waist and legs.

It is a dance when one posture is divided into three movements: one, da; two, da; three, da. When the three movements are combined into one, it is a knock-out technique.

When you have mastered the techniques of the two-person dance, you will know the functional use of the one hundred and fifty postures of T'ai Chi Ch'uan.

You say that when you practice alone it is important to imagine an opponent in front of you. Can you give an example of this?

Yes. For example, when practicing the posture, ''step forward, deflect downward, intercept and punch'', it should be followed by the ''withdraw and push'' posture. With these two postures you presume that an opponent strikes to your chest with his right fist. You neutralize this by placing your right wrist, palm up, on his right wrist. Then place your left palm, facing downward, on the inside of his right forearm and press it downward. This is called ''deflect''. Next, step forward with your left foot and at the same time move your left arm to the front and left side. This is called ''intercept.'' Proceed to strike his chest, using your right fist, with the ''tiger mouth'' facing upward. This is called ''punch.'' These are the three movements.

The second posture is called ''withdraw and push.'' The opponent seizes your right wrist as you strike out at his chest and he pushes it to the left. He does this with his left hand. You restore your body, crossing both hands together, with the palms facing the body. This is called ''withdraw.'' Secondly, separate your palms and turn them outward. With your right hand lightly touching his right wrist, push forward with both hands using the whole body as one unit. This is called ''push.''

This is the only way to practice T'ai Chi Ch'uan. If you have nothing in your mind in which to base your practice, your forms will gradually and unconsciously change. The functional uses of T'ai Chi will eventually be lost. Prof. Cheng Man-ch'ing told us this often. He said, "When practicing T'ai Chi singly, you must imagine that there is an opponent in front of you. This is one of the secret techniques I learned from the Yang family." It is very important that you do this.

Can you tell us exactly what you mean by the Three Treasures: ching, ch'i and shen?

The Chinese call the three treasures "san pao." Ching is the sperm, the sexual secretions of both the male and female. Ch'i (life giving principle) is a kind of oxygen in the body necessary for stamina and vitality. Shen is the spirit of vitality.

These three energies are within your person. They transfer from one to another. The ching will transfer to ch'i and the ch'i to shen. They rotate inside the body making one stronger and stronger. If the ching is weak or lost, that person will be sick. By practicing T'ai Chi Ch'uan, you will mobilize your energy so that the ching can be transferred into ch'i and from the ch'i into shen.

When a person is young and strong, the sperm is abundant. In an old man it is exhausted. Even if the sperm is abundant, though, trouble may come if one does not transfer it into ch'i. This "ching" or sexual secretion is not the same as the similar term used for intrinsic energy. Both words transliterate the same but are entirely different in meaning. When the ch'i is full, it likewise must be transferred into shen, the spirit of vitality. All three energies must transfer from one to another if one is to enjoy good health.

The spirit of vitality is expressed in your eyes. If it is strong, it is possible to see for a great distance. If it is weak, one can see only a few feet away. Eventually, that person will see nothing at all. When the three treasures are strong, one will be in perfect health.

What do you mean by "transferring?"

To transfer means to change. The Taoist's say, "lien ching wai ch'i" which means to "cultivate the sperm and transfer it into ch'i." Ching is the sperm and it is necessary to stimulate it. The best method to acommplish this is by practicing T'ai Chi Ch'uan. Gradually the ching will transfer into ch'i and the ch'i will penetrate the bones and become marrow. All three energies will return to their normal level as they are closely connected to one another. Animals are able to do this naturally. A tiger, for example, is very strong because the ch'i has penetrated the bone naturally and has turned into marrow. When the bones are full with marrow, they are very strong.

In the T'ai Chi classics it says, "suspend the head from above as if being held up by a string" or "retain a light and sensitive energy on top of the head." These are both ways in which to stimulate the spirit of vitality. It also says in the classics, "When the lowest vertebrae are plumb erect, the spirit of vitality reaches the top of head. With the top of the head suspended from above, as if by a thread, the whole body will feel light and nimble." This means that the practice of T'ai Chi Ch'uan is very good for a person's health because the spirit of vitality will become very strong.

It seems that there is a strong relationship between ch'i and intrinsic energy. Would you explain this?

To strike with the ch'i is to use intrinsic energy. It is important to exhale during the strike as this will allow the ch'i inside to come out. Without intrinsic energy the ch'i will just sit inside because it cannot get out by itself.

Suppose that during the strike, you inhale instead of exhale. This will be injurious because the ch'i will remain inside. If, however, you exhale when striking, the strike will be much more effective. Ch'i, when combined with the ching is very powerful.

When you strike someone, the opponent will feel the intrinsic energy only and not the ch'i. The person performing the strike will feel only his ch'i and not the intrinsic energy. They are closely connected.

So breathing is important here too?

Yes. I will give a few examples of breathing properly and explain how effective it is, if done correctly. The first one, I mentioned already, about exhaling when striking someone. But, suppose that your opponent is stronger than you and his energy comes back at you. Let's say he even pushes you over. Even though you fall, you will not be hurt unless you were inhaling as it happened. If you hold your breath when striking, you will be like a piece of wood, strong but not pliable. When you fall it is like one hard thing hitting another and you will be hurt. If you exhale, your body will be relaxed and flexible and little injury will occur. Children are like this. They are very soft and relaxed and when a child falls, it is rarely hurt. This is important when you are being pushed over. Do not tense up or the result will be worse.

When confronted by a man who is superior in skill, try to relax. It is difficult but necessary because if you tense up, you will do poorly. The psychological aspect of a confrontation is significant. You must keep your body under control.

In your book you discuss former heaven ch'i and early heaven ch'i. What do you mean by these two terms and how do they relate to T'ai Chi Ch'uan practice?

These terms mean the ch'i before heaven and after heaven. Although they are different, the result of each is the same. When practicing some will do it the way of "hsien tien hsi" and others by the method of "hou tien hsi". These terms mean reverse breathing and natural breathing, respectively.

Natural breathing, hou tien hsi, is the method in which the stomach becomes larger when the person inhales. When exhaling, it contracts and becomes smaller.

A great number of people that practice T'ai Chi Ch'uan use hsien tien hsi or reverse breathing. With reverse breathing, the stomach contracts as the person breathes in. Breathing out, it expands. With this type of breathing, one can acquire the art faster than by using the natural method but the final result is the same. Both methods are good. Which one you use is up to you. I prefer the hou tien hsi because it is the more natural way.

Some schools of T'ai Chi talk about the upper and lower tan–tien, the "third eye" and navel areas, calling it upper and lower level ch'i. What relationship do these have with former heaven ch'i and early heaven ch'i?

These things have nothing to do with the T'ai Chi way of breathing. When you exhale, the ch'i comes from the tan-tien which is one and one-third inches below the navel. The ch'i is stored here and it is from this area that it flows throughout the body. It does not come from the head. This is not the T'ai Chi way of practice.

When we practice T'ai Chi, how should we breathe and what is the role of breathing in T'ai Chi Ch'uan?

First let's discuss what a beginner must remember when practicing. A beginner must know the name of the posture, what direction to face, the number of beats and many other things. This will be done breathing naturally and without music. Eventually the beginner will do everything to the music. If, however, the person forgets the music, the breath will be used as a guide, that is, breathing will be used to control the beats. On the first beat, there is an inhalation, on the second beat, an exhalation, on the third, an inhalation and on the fourth, and exhalation. An exhale should always occur on the last beat of the posture. If this is done properly, over time it will be mastered both physically and mentally.

When a person can perform the postures with or without music with nothing in their mind, they have reached the highest level. The exercise may take twenty minutes or more. The method one has learned is forgotten and even the breathing. It is done naturally, without thought, with the mind absolutely empty. The person will feel as if in a trance and when finished they will wonder what it was they did and where they were. This stage where the mind is totally empty is very good for health.

When you talk about breathing, are you saying that the breath should be even in regards to the inhalation and the exhalation? Should not the exhalation be longer than the inhalation?

Yes. I have had many teachers and most of them advocated that when breathing, the exhalation be longer than the inhalation. Therefore, the inhalation is a bit quicker. It is the method I prefer.

How important is the practice of pushing-hands to T'ai Chi Ch'uan?

If you only practice the solo forms you will gradually acquire a root or central equilibrium. This is very important but you will never be able to interpret the strength of your opponent if you do not do two-person drills like pushing-hands.

Pushing-hands practice is necessary for learning self-defense skills. You will learn how to find a person's yin and yang aspects and locate his center of gravity. Every person is different. You will learn not to be double-weighted when you confront an opponent. Also you will learn to find the opponent's line of attack so you can push him over easily.

If you do not practice pushing-hands, you will not learn these things. It is necessary to use your hand to interpret and solo drills will not teach you this. I believe that a person cannot acquire a high level of skill if they do not practice pushing-hands.

One last question, sir?

How many last questions?

This is it. If T. T. Liang had one wish, what would it be?

I wish that all my students will become better than I. That is my wish. I wish also that everyone would practice T'ai Chi Ch'uan because it is an exercise for all people, the sick, young and old. Attaining this will be very difficult. It is all up to you.

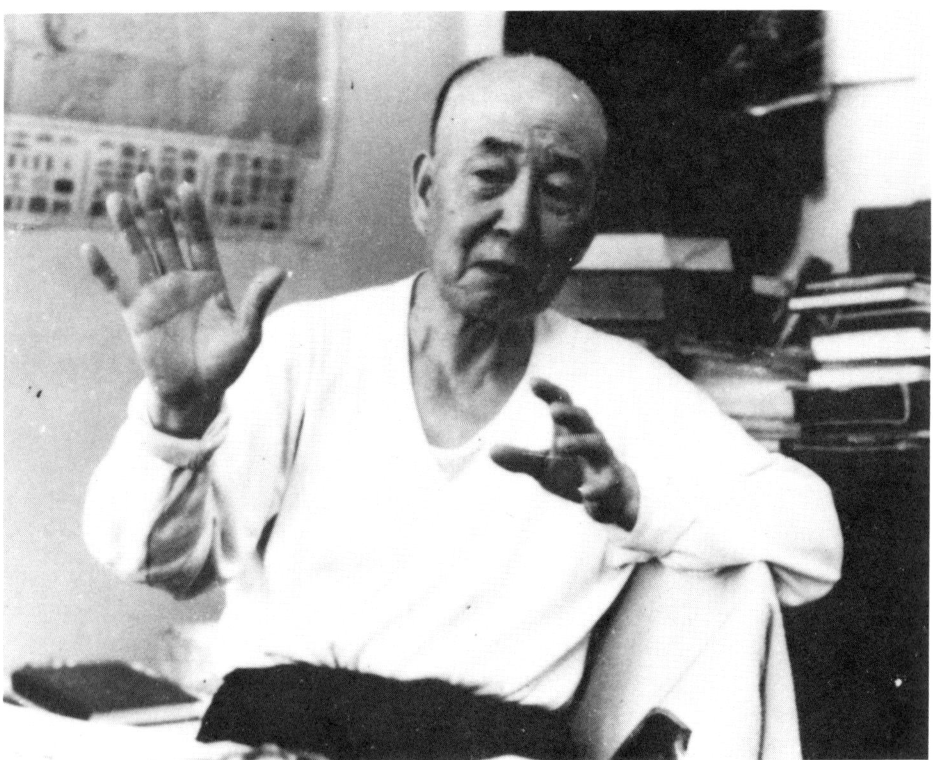

Chapter Two

Writings and Translations by Master T. T. Liang

Anecdotes of the Yang Family

Within the Chinese martial arts there are numerous categories and styles. Among them all, only the Wu-Tang school of T'ai Chi Ch'uan, handed down by the Taoist saint, Chang San-feng, is the pure internal system of these martial art varieties. Only through the method of relaxing the whole body, without exerting the slightest external muscular force, will the intrinsic energy be developed. This is the fundamental principle of the Wu-Tang school of T'ai Chi Ch'uan.

Yang Lu-chan, a native of Kuang Ping in Hopei province, received his T'ai Chi instruction from Chen Chang-hsing of Honan province. Yang Lu-chan handed down his art to his two sons, Pan-hou and Chien-hou, and Chien-hou to his sons, Shao-hou and Cheng-fu. The following is a general account of the anecdotes of the Yang family and their disciples. It is according to what had been recorded about this illustrious family.

Yang Lu-chan had learned the external system of martial art (like the hard style as Shaolin Boxing). Later he learned of Chen Chang-hsing, a native of Chen Chia Kuo (Chen family village) of Hwai Ching Prefecture in Honan province. Chen Chang-hsing was well versed in T'ai Chi Ch'uan, an internal system of martial art. Yang Lu-chan took all the money he had and travelled to Honan province to learn from Chen Chang-hsing.

Although he studied for several years, he was always defeated when testing himself with his fellow students. One night he got up to urinate and heard a strange sound coming from the other side of the wall. He climbed over it to find out what was happening. He saw that all his fellow students were gathered inside the great hall and that the teacher was explaining and demonstrating all the secret principles and techniques of T'ai Chi. Yang Lu-chan then concealed himself outside the window of the hall and watched. On returning to his room he practiced diligently what he could remember. Henceforth, he went to watch them every night without fail.

After a period of time, when some of his fellow students forced him to contest, Yang Lu-chan had no alternative but to consent, with the result that no one could overcome him. All his fellow students were astonished. His teacher then called Yang Lu-chan and said, ''I have examined you for several years and found you are an honest and sincere young man, with much patience, so I will, in person, show you the real meaning of T'ai Chi Ch'uan. Come to my room tomorrow.''

The next day he went to see his teacher and found him sitting in his chair napping, bobbing his head in a very uncomfortable manner. Yang Lu-chan stood quietly by his side for a long time but his teacher did not wake up. Thereupon, he supported his teacher's head with his hands for such a long time that he felt as though his arms were breaking. He dared not move at all. When his teacher finally awakened, he said, ''You are already here. I was tired and fell asleep. Come again tomorrow.'' Lu-chan left. The next day he went back at the appointed time and again found his teacher fast asleep. Lu-chan waited with bated breath. His teacher occasionally opened his eyes. Seeing Lu-chan standing there waiting calmly by his side, without any expression of hatred, he again said, ''Come back tomorrow.'' When Lu-chan arrived on the third day, his teacher said, ''This young man is worth teaching.'' From that day he taught Lu-chan the secrets of Chen's T'ai Chi and ordered him to practice when he returned home. Afterwards, whenever Lu-chan engaged in a contest with his fellow students, no one could overcome him. He was second to none.

One day, as Lu-chan was preparing to return to his home town, his teacher summoned everyone to meet together in the hall. Pointing to all of his own family disciples, he said, ''I have taught all of you the secrets of T'ai Chi and none of you have acquired it.'' Next, pointing to Lu-chan, he said, ''But I reluctantly gave my art to this man. Although he is not of our Chen clan, he, nonetheless, has obtained the essence of my art. He is now leaving.'' After Yang Lu-chan had filled his ambitions to the utmost, he returned home.

Lu-chan returned home penniless. Someone recommended him to teach at a rich family's home in the capital (Beijing). The rich family had already engaged one boxing teacher, whose martial skill was mediocre at best. This teacher became very jealous when Lu-chan came to teach in the same place. The jealous man insisted on a duel with Lu-chan. Lu-chan said, ''If you really want to fight, please inform the head of the family first.'' He did so and the host agreed, but said, ''I hope you both will take it as a friendly match; that you will set limits and not cause injury or death.'' Lu-chan arrived in the arena and stood erect without moving.The jealous teacher then suddenly extended his fist to hit Lu-chan with all his might. Without even seeing Lu-chan lift his hands, the jealous teacher was thrown more than ten feet away. The host was greatly surprised. He bowed in deep respect and said, ''I did not know that the level of your art was so profound and abstruse and was of such a high degree.'' Thereupon, he spread a sumptuous feast to honor him. After the banquet Lu-chan packed up and resigned his post. He then settled down within the capital city and taught Yang style T'ai Chi. So the people learning T'ai Chi in the capital were all Yang's disciples.

Yang Lu-chan handed down his art of T'ai Chi to his two sons, Pan-hou and Chien-hou. He expected his sons to acquire his art as quickly as possible, admonishing them to practice day and night without rest. While Pan-hou and Chien-hou were under their father's supervision, they met with unbearable treatment in their training. Pan-hou attempted to run away from home but was intercepted and brought home. Chien-hou even once tried to hang himself but was rescued in the nick of time.

Though they had not yet reached the age of twenty, they were already well known for their talent and ability. Their reputations were held high all over the capital. A nobleman heard of them and engaged Pan-hou as an instructor, offering him forty dollars per month salary. He showed Pan-hou great respect and bestowed honors upon him.

Mr. Liu of Hsiung Hsien practiced, "Yueh's irregular postures". He was of great strength, being capable of raising more than 500 pounds and had more than one thousand students learning from him. Somebody provoked hostilities on both sides. Pan-hou, who was a proud man, was unable to endure this provocation. He challenged Mr. Liu to a duel, which was to take place in the east city. The news spread throughout the capital and several thousand spectators gathered at the arena. After much of the crowd arrived, Mr. Liu immediately stretched out his hand and grasped Pan-hou's wrist tightly. Pan-hou applied the technique of, "intercepting energy to shake off and attack" which caused Mr. Liu to fall. He immediately left in great distress. As a result of the contest, Pan-hou's reputation spread far and wide; his name was held in high esteem on both sides.

When he returned home to see his father, he was elated with his victory. With a look of exultation, he gave a detailed account of how he knocked down Mr. Liu. His father gave a cold-hearted laugh and said, "Your strike was good enough but half your sleeve has been torn away. Is this called T'ai Chi?" Pan-hou looked down at his sleeve and found it was indeed the truth. He was downcast and left the house. He then recalled that when Mr. Liu had seized his wrist, it was like a dog's bite. After having received such a shock he practiced T'ai Chi more diligently than ever in order to improve himself.

Yang Cheng-fu said that his uncle, Yang Pan-hou, had a disciple named Fu Erh-yeh who lived at Chao Mien Lane in the east city. He was over seventy years of age but his appearance was that of a man in his fifties. His son was fifty some years old and everyone thought that they were brothers. Fu Erh-yeh commented, "Though I am the disciple of Yang Pan-hou, I am unable to hand down his art for I have not practiced in more than thirty years. My father did not allow me to practice T'ai Chi for this reason. Formerly, my elder brother learned the art of wrestling diligently without intermission. After several years he returned home. As soon as he saw me he asked, "How is your wrestling technique?" I told him I had not practiced it for a long time. I told him that I had learned T'ai Chi Ch'uan from Yang Pan-hou, who taught me how to relax and use the internal intrinsic energy and not the external muscular force. I said he also taught me how to neutralize an opponent's strength. My brother ridiculed me and would not believe in it whatsoever, so he struck out his fist to hit me. I used the T'ai Chi posture "Deflect Downward, Intercept and Punch" to counterattack. Unexpectedly my brother fell away through the hall to the outside yard. He lay on the ground face up and he could not get up, having been injured by the fall. He rested for several days and began to recover. I was severely reprimanded by my father and not allowed to practice T'ai Chi from then on. How pitiable it was, simply because I was too young and reckless."

Fu Erh-yeh continued his story. "My teacher's father, Yang Lu-chan, was fond of me, owing to my diligence and carefulness. I often stood at his side to serve him and fill his pipe with tobacco. At age eighty, Yang Lu-chan still vigorously practiced T'ai Chi Ch'uan daily without intermission. Occasionally he came to my house to chat. On one of these visits it was raining and the road was full of mud. When he arrived, I noticed that the soles of his shoes were white and clean as if they never touched the mud. They were without a speck of dirt. This is called, "the technique of treading on the snow without trace of a footstep." This is possible because the body of a T'ai Chi master is so light and nimble that he can raise his body up. When this is practiced to the highest level, he can raise his body up and walk in the air. Pan-hou had also acquired this technique but very few knew of it. I saw it only once.

Yang Lu-chan summoned his senior disciples by letter, asking them all to come to his house on a certain day. He intended to travel and he had some words of instruction for them. They all arrived at the appointed time but they thought something was strange because there was no cart ready outside the gate. When they went inside, they saw their teacher (Lu-chan) seated in the middle of the great hall. After all the disciples saluted him, each one helped fill his pipe with tobacco and then stood quietly by his side. Lu-chan called them one by one and spoke words of encouragement to them. He talked to them about the general principles of T'ai Chi. After a little while, Lu-chan suddenly brushed his sleeves, sat erect and passed away. After his death, his coffin was put in a monastery outside Chi Hua gate.

The monastery's five main halls faced south. On the east and west sides there were several sub-rooms. The coffin rested in the west sub-hall. Yang Pan-hou and his brother, Chien-hou, all lived in the west sub-hall. I also lived there so that I could serve them.

Later a southerner arrived at the monastery. He had very long fingernails and his speech was slurred. No one knew who he was, nor could they understand his words. One day my teacher came out from his room and said to me, 'Don't go out from this gate and do not talk with the southerner in the east sub-hall.' I promised I would not but wondered the reason why. At that time I was only nineteen and quite immature. When my teacher, Yang Pan-hou, left I stayed behind. I sat there quietly and after a period of time I needed to move about. I forgot the promise I had previously made to my teacher. I opened the gate and went into the main hall to play. In my right hand I held a cup full of tea and was spinning it around as I danced about. I jumped up onto a small table without spilling a drop. Just then I was seen by the southerner. He asked me questions about myself but I did not answer, as I remembered my teacher's order. I was frightened and returned to my own room.

The next day the chief monk of the monastery, who also knew the secret techniques of the martial arts quite well, had an earnest talk with Pan-hou. At first my teacher was troubled. I could see his face turn color. After a while he nodded his head and agreed to something. The monk went out and a little while later returned to my teacher, accompanied by the southerner. Pan-hou treated the southerner with unusual politeness. The three went out through the gate together. Later my teacher returned with a pleased look on his face. The southerner then packed up and left. No one ever said for sure, but considering all the mystery surrounding this southerner, I surmised that he was some form of a spirit body of Yang Lu-chan. This of course is just my opinion.

Yang Pan-hou had a daughter aged seventeen. She was a very beautiful and clever young lady whom my teacher loved very much. She died suddenly while he was away from home. When he heard the tragic news he immediately rushed home. The coffin, however, had already been closed. His pain and grief was so extreme over the loss of his beautiful daughter that his body suddenly raised off the floor seven to eight feet high, as if suspended in the air. The bystanders looked at him in awe. I had seen him do this on a few other occasions. He was capable of this as he had knowledge of the secret technique of levitation. His father, Yang Lu-chan, taught him this art. Pan-hou's pain was so extreme that without even realizing it, he disclosed his extraordinary technique and skill.''

Although the Yang brothers, Chien-hou and Pan-hou, were well versed in the martial art of T'ai Chi Ch'uan and were very well known, they usually kept their art secret and would not show it off. They especially knew how to control their tempers and had not the slightest intention of flaunting their supremacy. They were extraordinarily humble and modest. People not well acquainted with them often mistook them for fools. It is true, indeed, that great wisdom seems like folly and great valor appears as cowardice. So a man should not be judged solely by his appearance or mannerisms.

One year a southerner (Cantonese) came to visit with Yang Pan-hou who was then already over sixty years old. The southerner showed him great respect and in admiration said, ''I have heard that the sticking energy of T'ai Chi Ch'uan is excellent. It is like glue on the body and one is unable to get rid of it. I would sincerely like some instruction from you.'' Pan-hou replied, ''I have learned from my ancestor (Yang Lu-chan) and know only a little of this art. I really do not possess such talent as you describe.'' So the southerner's request was obstinately refused. But the southerner requested instruction over and over again. Pan-hou then said, ''I am sure that you are well versed in this art, but as old and worthless as I am, how can I compete with you?'' After a momentary pause, Pan-hou said, ''Please show me the method of test and let us see whether or not I can exert my strength in pursuit of the goal.'' The southerner happily responded, ''Let us try this. Take several tens of bricks that have been evenly placed in the yard with a distance of two feet between each one, like a T'ai Chi round form. We will both stand on the bricks. I will be in front and you will follow in back with your hand lightly touching my back. We start to walk round and round, like turning a mill, without letting our feet touch the ground. You must not let go of my back. If your feet touch the ground or if your hand gets away from my back, it will be considered a defeat.'' Pan-hou replied, ''Mill Turning Round Walking'' will easily make one giddy and I am afraid I won't be able to make it. But as long as you have raised the question, I cannot but obey your order and put forth my best effort to try my luck at this.'' So in the yard they started to arrange the bricks as the southerner had suggested. As soon as everything was in order, the southerner stepped onto the bricks, walking slowly in front and Pan-hou, sinking the ch'i to his tan-tien and concentrating his spirit of vitality within, followed behind with his hand lightly attached to the southerner's back for several rounds. The body of the southerner was light as a swallow and his steps grew faster and faster like a flying wheel. Pan-hou applied his 'Flying Upward To Chase The Wind And To Pursue The Lightning' technique to follow him, so that he would not separate from him. The southerner found that there was no way in which to get rid of Pan-hou, so he suddenly raised his body and flew up onto the roof of the house. He then turned his head, looked down into the courtyard and found no trace of Pan-hou. He was very frightened. But as he turned his head back again, he found Pan-hou was still behind him with his hand lightly touching his back as before. Pan-hou then said, ''You really made fun of me. I am tired now, why don't we get down and rest a little while?''

The southerner was greatly startled and could not but highly respect Pan-hou. They had made a warm friendship. The southerner later went on his way.

Yang Chien-hou was an instructor of the Shen Wu Battalion at the age of seventy. One day, on his way home, a coarse fellow took him by surprise and attacked him with a club from the rear. Chien-hou, with a sudden turn of his body, held the club with his hand and with a slight push, sent the man flying more than twenty feet.

Yang Chien-hou could hold a swallow in his palm without letting the bird fly away. A bird about to take off must first press downwards with its feet and find a firm foothold upon which to exert energy so as to raise its body aloft. Chien-hou could intercept the sinking energy of the bird's two claws. As the bird would push downwards, he would relax and neutralize; the swallow, unable to avail itself of a foothold, could not fly away. From this we can see the clever, subtle and ingenious use of intercepting and neutralizing energy that Chien-hou had acquired. No one else could approach his level of ability.

Yang Lu-chan had a disciple named Wang Lan-ting whose art of T'ai Chi was very profound. Unfortunately he died at a young age. It was heard that Wang Lan-ting had a disciple named Li Pin-fu who was also very skilled. Many people came to challenge him but no one could defeat him. Once a young person, who spoke with a southern accent, came to visit Li Pin-fu. The young person's hand was several inches away from a chair in the hall. Upon stretching out his hand, the chair immediately was raised up and suspended in the air. The young person wished to compete with Li Pin-fu but he modestly declined. The young man insisted. It just so happened that Li Pin-fu was holding a puppy under his left arm. He could only parry with his right arm but after several turns of his body, Li Pin-fu caused the young person to fall. Weeping bitterly, the young man left defeated. He had great skill but could not fight well.

An Essay On The Essentials Of T'ai Chi Ch'uan

The theories behind T'ai Chi Ch'uan (often simply called T'ai Chi) are not easy to comprehend because of their depth and subtlety. The techniques, moreover, are quite difficult to acquire. The correct method is of the utmost importance. One must learn things in proper sequence and allow progress to come in a gradual and natural manner, otherwise, studying for an entire lifetime will be to no avail. In the ''Song of Thirteen Postures'' it says, ''Pay special attention to your every posture and seek out its hidden meaning, then you can acquire this art without exerting excessive effort.''

There are three important T'ai Chi ''Classics.'' The first one, called the T'ai Chi Ch'uan Classic, was handed down by Chang San-feng, a Taoist of the late Sung dynasty. This classic begins by saying, ''In every movement the entire body should be light and agile and all of its parts connected like a string of pearls.'' The opposite of light and agile is heavy and clumsy and the opposite of connected like a string of pearls is dispersed and confused. This indicates the coordination of substantial and insubstantial and discloses the objective of the fundamental principle of T'ai Chi.

It goes on to say, ''The ch'i should be stimulated and the spirit of vitality should be concealed within.'' This again emphasizes the importance of the internal cultivation of ch'i and spirit of vitality.

The classic continues, ''There should be no deficiency and no excess, no hollows, no projections, no severance and no splice.'' These defects result from using external muscular force. If, however, the mind-intent is employed to direct the movements of the body, the entire body will be relaxed and pliable so as to fulfill the requirement of being ''light and agile, its parts connected like a string of pearls.''

Again it says, ''the energy is rooted in the feet, developed in the legs, directed by the waist and moved up to the fingers. The feet, legs and waist must act as one so that when advancing and retreating, you will obtain a good opportunity and a superior position.'' The above explains the systematic method of practice.

These three paragraphs, all discussing the classic handed down by Chang San-feng, have revealed the important points of the principles, methods and functions. The principles indicate the reason why; the methods indicate what ought to be and the functions reveal the efficacy of both the principles and methods. These three are all interdependent and mutually supportive of each other in practice. Not one of them should be lacking. By practicing in this way, one will accord with what is called, ''the unification of civil and martial aspects; the equal importance of principle and technique and the combined cultivation of external and internal.''

T'ai Chi Ch'uan is a combination of civil and martial aspects. The civil aspect stresses principles and the martial stresses techniques. Both must be taken into account; neglecting either one is not real T'ai Chi.

The civil aspect is called Tao (principles) and the martial aspect is called skill (techniques). Tao emphasizes internal cultivation; skill emphasizes external development. Cultivating ones nature (temperament) is called internal development and training the muscles and bones is called external development. Both are important and neither can be lacking. So we can see that the unification of both civil and martial aspects, the equal importance of Tao and skill and the combination of internal cultivation with external training is the very best method for beginners to learn T'ai Chi Ch'uan.

When one practices T'ai Chi, it is important to direct all the movements of mind-intent. As the ''Song of the True Interpretation of T'ai Chi'' says, ''formless and imageless (forgetting oneself), the whole body completely relaxed (internal and external united into one) and forgetful of everything, returning to the natural way (following the desire of the mind) . . . '' This indicates the mind-intent has reached the ultimate stage.

The T'ai Chi classic states, ''The movements of upward and downward, backward and foreward, left and right are to be directed by the mind-intent and not by external muscular force.'' The mind-intent refers to the internal spiritual function and the outer aspect refers to the movements of the postures motivated by external muscular force. If every movement can be directed by the mind-intent within and manifested without, the internal spiritual aspect and external physical aspect will be united. Upper and lower parts of the body will move in unison. The body will instantly follow the dictates of the mind and the ch'i and intrinsic energy will immediately reach the intended point.

It is evident that, at the beginning, if you try to use mind-intent to direct the movements, your skill will be improved by leaps and bounds. Gradually when you have mastered the use of your mind, you will be able to acquire all the techniques. Therefore, the most important guiding point of T'ai Chi Ch'uan is the use of mind-intent to direct the movements. If one can take hold of this important point and constantly comprehend the principles, one will obtain the very essence of T'ai Chi. As the T'ai Chi classics say, "The more you practice, the more you will master the art. By silently remembering and thoroughly comprehending, you will eventually reach a state of complete reliance on the mind."

The second important treatise was written by Wang Chung-yueh of the Ming dynasty. In the beginning it says, "T'ai Chi (Supreme Ultimate) evolved from Wu Chi (infinity) and is the mother of yin and yang. In movement, the two become separated; in stillness, they combine into one. There should be no excess and no insufficiency. You yield as the opponent stretches out." The above indicates that T'ai Chi was derived from the principles of the I Ching.

The treatise then says, "To conquer the strong by yielding is called withdrawal; to make a favorable position of your own and a defective one of your opponent's, is termed adherance. You respond quickly to fast action and respond to slow action in a leisurely manner. Although the changes are numerous, the principle is the same (that of an all prevading unity)." The above includes all the principles and techniques of T'ai Chi.

The third treatise is Wang Chung-yueh's, "Mental Elucidation of the Thirteen Postures." It emphasizes especially the methods of practice with the utmost delicacy and accuracy. In the beginning this treatise states, "Let the mind direct the ch'i . . . " "Mind" here refers to mind-intent, which is a human perception. This is the leading principle of the entire treatise. It goes on to say, "The mind is the commander, the ch'i is the flag and the waist is the banner." Also, "The mind leads and the body follows . . . when performing all of the movements, one's mind-intent is directed to the spirit of vitality and not to the external use of breath or physical force." These phrases all indicate the importance of mind-intent when practicing T'ai Chi.

The above three treatises include all the essential aspects of T'ai Chi Ch'uan, omitting none. Students must make a thorough investigation of them and comprehend deeply their meaning in order to acquire this art.

Discriminating The Process of Attainment Of T'ai Chi Ch'uan

The general outline of the T'ai Chi Ch'uan exercise is divided into three levels: Man, Earth and Heaven. The lowest level, Man, is an exercise to relax the sinews and circulate the blood. It is subdivided into three steps. The first step is to relax the sinews from the shoulders to the fingers, the second step is to relax the sinews from the thighs to the bubbling-well points and the third step is to relax the sinews from the lowest vertebrae to the pai hui (crown).

The middle level, Earth, is an exercise to open and penetrate into articulations of the joints. It is subdivided into three steps. The first step is to sink the ch'i to the tan-tien, the second step is to penetrate the ch'i to the bubbling-well points and the third step is to penetrate the ch'i to the pai hui point.

The highest level, Heaven is an exercise of the functions of perception: It is subdivided into three steps. The first step is to "hear" or try to find out by listening to the energy. The second step is to comprehend the energy. The third step is to arrive at a complete mastery of your opponent. This is a divinely intelligent energy. So there are altogether three levels and nine steps. I will explain them one by one in detail.

Man

The method of the first step of Man's level is to relax the sinews from the shoulders to the fingers. If one can relax the sinews, the blood will be naturally active and lively. The process is to relax the sinews of the wrists first, then the elbows and then the shoulders. Without exerting the slightest external muscular force the whole body should be completely relaxed and the movements should be as flexible as possible. Throughout all the movements one has to seek the straight from the bent and imitate the round form. Too much bending or straightness are both incorrect. There should be neither deficiency nor excess, neither hollows or projections. In the end one must achieve relaxation of the sinews to the middle fingers. This is the first step of Man's level.

The second step of Man's level is to relax the sinews from the thighs to the heels of the feet. The processes are the same as the first step but the difference is that the light and heavy, empty and solid must be clearly discriminated. The feet are capable of supporting the whole body's weight. It is different from the movements of the hands which are easy and convenient. Ordinarily we never pay attention to the substantial and insubstantial of the feet and even martial arts boxers let them take their own course. In T'ai Chi Ch'uan the weight must be put on one foot when the other foot is ready to move forward or backward. It is not allowed to use the slightest muscular force. The thighs, the knees and the heels should be soft and relaxed; the weight should be on the bubbling-well points which are attached to the ground. So the substantial and insubstantial of the feet must be clearly discriminated. It is likewise with the hands. The only difference is that when the right foot is substantial, the right must be insubstantial. If this is not the case, it is double-weighting, which should be absolutely avoided from the T'ai Chi point of view. So this is called the second step of Man's level.

The third step of Man's level is to relax the sinews from the lowest vertebrae to the top of the head. The processes are the same as the first step. The spine is the main bone of the body and is its support. It has many joints. It is said that a soft waist will bend as though boneless. From this we can see that the spine must also be flexible. The flexibility of sinews relies upon their softness. The most important thing is that the lowest vertebrae must be plumb erect and the top of the head held as if suspended from above. This is called the third step of Man's level.

Earth

The first step of Earth's level is to sink the ch'i to the tan-tien which is the preliminary foundation of imbibing energy. The tan-tien is situated about 1⅓ inches below the navel. By dividing a horizontal line joining the navel and spine into a ratio of 3:7, measuring from the navel, the tan-tien is found. The mind and ch'i abide by the tan-tien and gradually the ch'i will be nourished. All should be carried out in a natural manner and should not have the slightest forced interpretation.

It is not easy for beginners to learn how to sink the ch'i to the tan-tien. It is necessary to drop the shoulders and lower the elbows. The chest must be slightly concave and the back a little bent. In this way one can cause the ch'i to sink to the tan-tien. Contrary to this, the ch'i will suddenly go up, the shoulders will be raised and the lungs will be lifted up. This manner of holding the body makes it easy for disease to enter.

When the ch'i sinks to the tan-tien it will reach to the four limbs. The ch'i should be directed by the mind so that it will reach the thighs, knees, heels, and the shoulders, elbows and wrists. When the joints of the four limbs are all open, the ch'i can pass downward to the bubbling-well points and upward to the pai hui point and finally to the tips of the middle fingers. The T'ai Chi Classics say, "When the mind directs the ch'i to circulate freely through the whole body, then one can devote oneself to the art of T'ai Chi." This is the second step of the Earth level.

When the ch'i passes over the lowest vertebrae and reaches to the pai hui point, it is called, "passing through three barriers." To pass the ch'i over the lowest vertebrae is the most difficult barrier; the first and second barrier are much easier. When you have practiced T'ai Chi for a long time, according to the correct way, your art will reach a higher level and your ch'i will naturally pass the lowest vertebrae. There should not be the slightest constraint, otherwise it will be in vain and also cause disease. Great caution is to be taken. When the ch'i passes the lowest vertebrae, penetrates into the spine, crosses over the occiput and finally reaches the crown, you have entered the door, that is, you have acquired the correct way of T'ai Chi. It not only can ward off disease and prolong life but is also a short way to achieving Immortality. This is the third step of the Earth level.

Heaven

We have to hear the energy. What is energy? How can we hear it? We have to examine these questions minutely. Now let me explain in detail. There is a big difference between energy and force. A secret handed down by the ancient T'ai Chi masters says, "Energy is from the sinews and tendons, whereas, force is from the bones." True indeed is this saying.

It is called energy because the ch'i issued from the sinews and tendons is flexible and elastic. Only by being flexible can one adhere, join, stick to and follow the opponent. By adhering and joining, my ch'i will come in contact with the ch'i of the opponent and so test the motion and tranquility of his ch'i. Therefore, we say "to hear." If your opponent does not move, you do not move. At his slightest stir you have already anticipated it and moved beforehand, taking the opportunity to attack him. This is called the function of sensation. It is the first step of the Heaven level.

We have to understand the energy. The difference between understanding the energy and hearing the energy is like the difference between the deep and shallow and the fine and the coarse. If the opponent stirs only slightly, I can hear it so I move first but to move first I must understand the energy. To obtain a superior posture of your own and to put your opponent in a defective position, this matter rests with yourself and not with your opponent. This is from the shallow to the profound.

It is rather more difficult to describe from coarse to fine. The T'ai Chi classics handed down by the ancient masters say, "When the opponent stirs slightly, I know by hearing it." A slight stir of the opponent's body is easy to examine but if his body does not move, it is hard to understand. If you can hear and know that the opponent is completely still, then you will arrive at a complete mastery of your opponent. This is called, "divine intelligence."

The ch'i from the sinews, veins, membranes and diaphragm are divided into four kinds of energy:

1) defence
2) hidden (latent)
3) ready to issue
4) withdraw and attack

The sinews enable movement of the joints. The veins can circulate the blood. The membranes are attached between the muscles and the flesh and they wrap the bones and sinews. The bowels and viscera are also wrapped by the membranes.

The ch'i from the sinews will not lose its normal attitude. When the ch'i is from the sinews we know that he is going to defend himself. We know that he is going to remain hidden and produce variations when the ch'i is from the veins. When the ch'i is from the diaphragm, that means that he wants to concentrate the energy internally, to withdraw and attack. This is the height of understanding energy. It is ingenious. Nothing compares to it. This is the second step of the Heaven level, "divine intelligence."

If you pay attention to your spirit of vitality and ignore your ch'i, your striking power will be as strong as pure steel. If you only pay attention to your ch'i, your blood circulation will be impeded and your striking power will be inactive and inefficient. When you practice T'ai Chi slowly, effortlessly and continuously, without exerting the slightest external muscular force for a long time, your ch'i will be gradually transformed into spirit of vitality. The issue of the intrinsic energy from the spirit of vitality will be as strong as steel refined a hundred times over. There is no stiff adversary who cannot be overthrown. The ancient T'ai Chi masters could push a person more than thirty feet away without any visible movement of the hands or body and could also knock down a person with any part of their body. This is called supernatural power or divinely intelligent energy. The T'ai Chi Classics say, "From the mastery of all the postures you will apprehend interpreting energy. From apprehending interpreting energy, you will arrive at a complete mastery of your opponent. Without a long period of arduous practice you cannot find yourself suddenly possessed of this wide and far reaching insight."

Ordinarily we do not see the power in a black cloud passing in the air but if any creature clashes against it, the thunder and lightning hidden in the cloud will immediately burst out. The supernatural power of a T'ai Chi master functions the same way. This is the third step of the Heaven level. You have to ascend step by step and should not skip over any detail. I wish to follow the mind of Chang San-feng and Wang Chung-yeuh and accomplish the unfinished will of these two great T'ai Chi masters. T'ai Chi is the best way to make the race and the nation powerful and productive. I hope all people learning T'ai Chi will exert themselves.

Why I Adopted Music To T'ai Chi Ch'uan

More than one thousand years ago, a Chinese monk named, Chan Chung, developed a method of concentration during meditation. He told people to repeat silently, ''What did I look like before I was born?'', that is, ''What did I look like when I was in my mother's womb?'' Later this method was handed down to Japan as Zen Dao except they use the question, ''What is Mu (nothing)?''

We often say that a man's heart is like a monkey, jumping and turning around all the time and his mind is like a horse, galloping without pause. When a man begins to practice meditation, his heart and mind are fully occupied with short thoughts. When one thought is gone, it is immediately replaced by another, giving the heart and mind no chance to rest and concentrate. So monk, Chan Chung, used his way of concentration to cut out all of the other short, confused thoughts. As the question, ''What did I look like before I was born?'' can never be solved, you have to repeat it over and over again for a long time. Gradually your heart and mind will become peaceful and quiet. Only one thing will be left to think of — ''What did I look like before I was born?'' Finally you will forget even the words you are concentrating on, so your heart and mind will be empty; your body will be completely relaxed; the ch'i will sink and abide by the tan-tien and the blood will circulate through the whole body without hindrance. It is good for health and the way to metamorphose into a Buddha.

It is the same with practicing T'ai Chi. In T'ai Chi the ascent to the highest level is divided into four steps. They are:

1. When beginning the practice of T'ai Chi you will have to memorize the number of beats, the directions, the practical uses of each posture and the ten guiding points as described in my book, **''T'ai Chi Ch'uan for Health and Self-Defense.''** You will breathe naturally and you will not use music.
2. After you have attained a degree of mastery of the things mentioned above, you will begin to use the beats, music, and proper breathing (methods of inhaling and exhaling). The rest you will forget.
3. At the next stage you will use only the music for concentration.
4. After practicing T'ai Chi with music for a sufficient length of time, you will forget the music, the movements and even yourself, although, you will proceed as usual. At this stage you will be in a trance and your five attributes: form, perception, consciousness, action and knowledge, will be empty. This is complete relaxation of the body and mind. It is very good for health and the way to immortality.

Of course, if one can reach the highest level while practicing T'ai Chi without music, so much the better. I cannot do it because I am a human being, an ordinary, ignorant person with a heart like a monkey and mind like a horse. I must use music as a means of concentration, as a stepping stone to the highest level of T'ai Chi.

I like music, especially soft music. I believe it is in a human being's nature. It can relieve tension and anxiety, produce happiness and relaxation and increase harmony and coordination.

During the forty years I have practiced T'ai Chi to music, I have taught in many universities, colleges and high schools. I have had thousands of students study with me. They have said that T'ai Chi with music is more enjoyable than without it. T'ai Chi with music has value and is not extraneous to the essence of T'ai Chi Ch'uan. If it was, I would not be eighty-six years of age and enjoying perfect health. I like music and have chosen to continue practicing T'ai Chi to music to maintain my good health.

T'ai Chi Ch'uan

A lecture by Professor Cheng, Man-ch'ing
Recorded by Liang, Tung-tsai

Forward:

T'ai Chi is a phsyical exercise and art of self-defense, invented by the Taoist, Chang San-feng, five centuries ago. In this exercise one has to breathe naturally, relax the muscles of the whole body so as to gain the help of the circulation of "ch'i" and blood and keep the posture and movements in complete balance. Its main object is to prevent illness, to lengthen life and to strengthen one's body and mind. If this stage is accomplished one can seek the method of self-defence. Even if one hits me with great force, I have no fear of him because I can overcome him. When I first learned T'ai Chi Ch'uan, its original procedure consisted of 128 movements. This series required more than ten minutes to go through. For the sake of time saving, I cut off the repeated motions and deleted the similar ones to get thirty-six forms.These forms preserve the essence of the original postures. A practice of this form requires only three minutes in quick time and five minutes with slower movements. If one practices it once each morning and evening, it takes only ten minutes to complete.

I. The General Principles Of Exercise. There are but two objects for exercise. If it is not for the body, it is for its practical use. In order to realize these objects, one must consider the following six elements: (1) the duration of practice, (2) the degree of attainment, (3) the difference in energy used, (4) the range of changes, (5) the skill of application, and (6) the speed of comprehension. These six elements depend upon proper instruction, natural talent, and perseverence. Of the three conditions, the first and third are similarily important. Without proper instruction, even with natural talent and perseverence one will not be successful. If one cannot persevere, even if one possesses natural talent and has good instruction, it will be difficult to acquire the art.

The Classics say, "Sink the ch'i (breath) to the "tan-tien" (the pubic region) and spread it throughout the body. Operate ch'i by the will and operate the body by the ch'i so the bones become permeated with it." The extreme of this practice will be when a person can throttle their breath (ch'i), down to the softness of breath in a child. This kind of attainment comes from accumulation of ch'i which enables an accumulation of strength and the energy produced will be inestimable. It all depends upon the method of instruction and the depth of knowledge.

However, by what way does one proceed to learn? The primary requirement is relaxation. One has to relax the body completely and thoroughly so that the ch'i can run through the joints and muscles freely. With regards to ch'i, it has to be sunk to the "tan-t'ien" first. To do this, the bosom has to be kept open in order to let the ch'i sink down and gradually accumulate. This is the beginning of the accumulation of ch'i. That is called exercise. Exercise must be set in operation first before it is in motion. An automobile or steamboat must be operated by steam first before it can move. So the movements of hands and feet must first be mobilized by ch'i.

II. Principles In Regard To The Body. Statements in the classics say, "Keep the coccyx upright and centered so to make one's spirit pass upward to the top of the head. This will result in lightness and comfort of the whole body by having the head in an upright position as if hanging in the air." These discuss the main method of exercising the spinal column. If the head is hung on a beam it cannot move in any direction. The spinal column is strengthened because the spinal column from the coccyx upward to the head is controlled. Strengthening of the spinal column does not only give more strength to the viscera inside the body but also makes the brain more efficient. This is the function of repairing one's bodily essence.

Next in importance is the sinking of the ch'i to the "tan t'ien." The "tan t'ien" is a technical term used by the Taoists. It means symbolically a piece of land in which seeds are sown for the purpose of creating a sort of nutritious element called "tan" or elixir of immortality. Its position is beneath the naval by 1.3 inches, nearer to the navel than to the spine in a proportion of 3 to 7. If one's ch'i is abundant in the "tan t'ien" the membranes of the whole body will be strengthened. A membrane is just like the inner tube of a tire. When there is ample ch'i in the "tan t'ien", the skin will become tougher and therefore, able to resist impact.

III. Principles In Regard To The Use. The use of T'ai Chi Ch'uan depends upon understanding the essence of the principles. The necessity of "getting the chance and seizing the condition" and the application of "pulling four ounces of strength to ward off one thousand pounds of impact" teach the user to do of this form of defense with understanding and not by brute strength. Fighting originally relied upon the use of technique with boldness and strength. Having no boldness and no strength, technique alone accomplished nothing. But the idea of T'ai Chi Ch'uan is contrary to the usual concept. Both boldness and strength have to be abandoned. T'ai Chi requires, "a lithesome body in any movement" and for the motion to be so exact that, "a feature cannot be added to it and a fly cannot alight on it without setting it in motion."

The classics also tell the novice, "Abandon yourself and follow your opponent." Isn't it strange to learn to abandon oneself and to follow one's opponent as a means of defense? For instance, when one hits me with great impact, how can I yield myself and follow him? Such a thing seems to be unbelievable. When I am hit with powerful impact, I do not hit back but also do not resist his strike. However, I do not accept his strike either but send the impact back by following his striking force. In this way my opponent will fall down by the impact of his own strength. This is the way of getting the chance and warding off one thousand pounds of impact by the application of four ounces of my pull. It is derived from the principle of abandoning oneself to follow the opponent. The principle has to be understood figuratively. It does not mean to use a thing of four ounces to push back an impact of one thousand pounds in reality.

The exercise the novice should begin with is "tui shou." In this form of exercise one should follow the principle of four words: adhering, joining, touching, and following. Adhering means to stick together. Joining means not to let the hands fall apart. These two words point to the upward and downward movements. The other two words apply to the forward and backward and the right and left movements.

In this exercise one is told, ''not to abandon, nor push back violently.'' Not to abandon means not to resist the attack of the opponent. The hands of the opposing parties are pushing in circular motion by repetition, just like the inseparability of shadow from body or echo from sound. When this form of exercise has been practiced for a long time one can leave the force applied to rotate by itself, coming or going, ebbing or waning, increasing or decreasing, reinforcing and withdrawing and yielding or resisting. If such variations are felt, then the student can be said to have gained the primary principle of the technique. Through continual practice one will gradually comprehend the idea of force applied and will have reached the advanced stage.

IV. How Can The Roots Of The Opponent Be Pulled Up? In ''tui shou'', when energy is issued, it is most effective if the two heels of the opponent can be pulled up. If only the front part of the opponent's feet are pulled up, the method of pulling up and letting down is not accurate enough. To be able to pull up the opponent's two heels, the following six essentials should be observed.

1. The classics say, ''The root is one's feet and the force is sent out through the legs, controlled by the hips and operated by the fingers. From the feet upward through the legs to the hips, the movement should be executed as one whole.'' The idea is that when a force is sent out, one should stand with the hips slightly backward as if in a sitting posture. This will make use of the elasticity of the hind part of the thighs and hold the hips in the right position. The force sent out should have the tendency to raise something upward. The elasticity of the hind part of the thighs is shifted to the front, to make the force go into the ground, where the man stands. Bending of the knees should not project beyond the toes. If they do, the force issued will become loose. Only with square shoulders, downward extending arms, a straight spinal column and an upright head can the force of the whole body be sent out in unison so that no root cannot be pulled up. If some slight deviation arises in a certain part, the force will be greatly reduced.
2. When both hands touch the body of the opponent, the strength applied should never be too much, otherwise it will be felt by the opponent who will try to neutralize it. It will then be impossible to pull up his root.
3. When both hands touch the opponent's body, it is better to be able to feel the wavering in him. It is most effective to issue one's energy at the moment of the wavering signs of the opponent although it is difficult to feel the wavering of the opponent's body. This has to be learned by hard work in ''tui shou'' exercise.
4. In issuing one's energy, never do it with both hands simultaneously. If energy is sent out simultaneously by both hands, it is a double application. The classics say, ''Energy should be issued only on one side.'' So, application by both hands at the same time is contrary to the principle of one-sided application. It will be better to issue energy through one hand, with the other hand ready to help.

5. The distance between the body and the hands should remain unchanged before and after the sending out of energy. If, in issuing energy, the hands either stretch out or withdraw, it will influence the application of energy from one's body, in unison and decrease the effect of pulling up the root.
6. In issuing energy, both hips and thighs should be kept relaxed in a sitting position. Then, when the energy is actually being sent out, the body changes to a rising position to make the pulling up work possible. The classics say, "If one intends to rise up he should have the idea of sitting down. If he intends to lift a thing up, he should apply energy pushing it down first to shake the roots, so that they will break off by themselves." This is the very idea.

V. My Interpretation. Man has to have physical exercise. The Book of Change says, "The movement of heaven is full of power. Thus the superior man makes himself strong and untiring." That is the foundation of making oneself strong. Of the same reason, "a door pivot never get worm eaten and running water never becomes putrid." However, there are many ways of exercise. One has to make a choice. Some like weight lifting, wrestling, or running; others like playing ball, skating, swimming, boxing and some like fencing. Each man has his own taste. But all of them cannot get away from the principle of using strength and competing for speed. This does not apply to T'ai Chi Ch'uan. This form of exercise can be learned by the sick, the old, the young and the weaker sex because it does not require the use of much strength, nor does it require speed. If it is practiced by youth or adults it will not have the effect of promoting indiscreet fighting or of seeking to overpower others. It can be enjoyed in any kind of weather, rain or shine, hot or cold. It can be practiced in any kind of environment, disregarding whatever kind of profession one engages in. It meets no danger as in skating or swimming. It requires little strenuous work as in boxing, wrestling and fencing. Only an area of three square feet and a short interval of seven minutes are required. So long as one has the mind to learn, one does not have to spend a cent to perform the exercise.

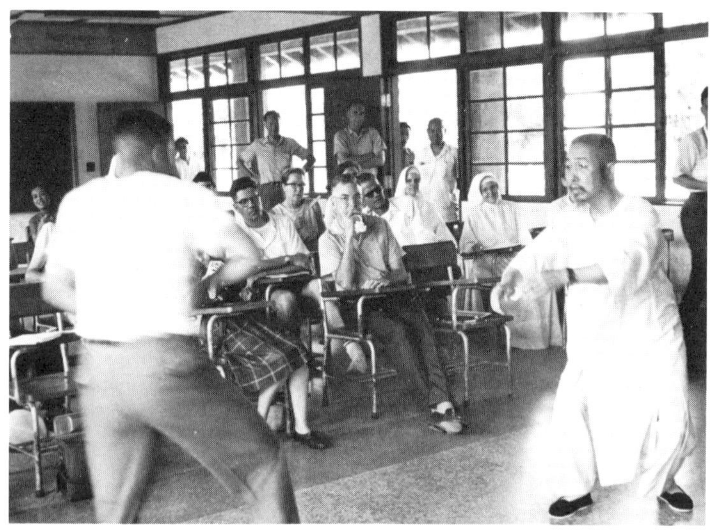

Chapter Three
T'AI CHI CH'UAN
Form Instructions

Yang Style Long Form
150 Postures

Arranged by Master T'ung–Tsai Liang

The following instructions for these 150 postures were taken from Master Liang's original notes which he composed more than ten years prior to this printing. In some cases there are a few minor variations concerning the execution of a posture. Ten years have passed and like all things there has occured change. These variations, however are neither frequent nor drastic enough to summon detailed comment here. Besides, the purpose of this work is not to decide nor argue at which time in Master Liang's career he was more correct in his teachings, as that would be a great error in itself. Therefore, it was decided to present the instructions as Master Liang originally composed them. Otherwise I fear misinterpretation because everyone, myself included, see the same thing a little differently.

Comp., S.A.O.

Acknowledgements:

Many thanks to Master Liang for appearing in the posture photographs of the form section and to Jonathan Russell for the photographs depicting the individual beats.

Key

Right Toe Movements:

Rt. Toe In 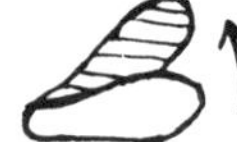 Rt. Toe Out 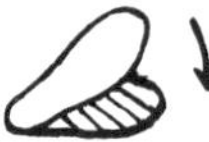

Left Toe Movements:

Lt. Toe In 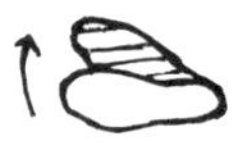 Lt. Toe Out 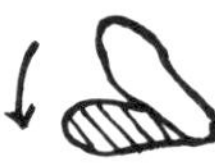

The majority of the toe ins and toe outs are 45 degrees, however, some are less, like "Lifting Hands" and some are more, like "Squatting Single Whip."

Toe 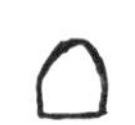 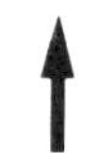 Heel 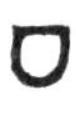

Weight Distributions:

All numbers are percentages. Therefore, a distribution of 70R-30L means:
70 percent of weight on the right foot
30 percent of weight on the left foot

Wu Chi

Before actually beginning the movements of T'ai Chi one stands in the Wu Chi posture. This posture, however, is not counted as one of the 150 postures of the form itself because there is no movement; yin and yang have not yet separated. The principles of this posture are as follows:

- Suspend the head as if by a thread from above.
- Gaze levelly to the front.
- Lower the shoulders.
- Hollow the chest.
- Hold the spine erect.
- Hang the arms downward and loosely along the sides of the body.
- Draw in the buttocks.
- Sink the ch'i to the tan-tien.
- Bend the knees slightly (do not lock the knee joints).
- With heels of both feet touching separate the toes so to form a "V" shape with the feet.
- Place the tongue on the roof of the mouth, lightly close the teeth and lips and stand quietly until all the tension in the body disappears.

Wu Chi in translation means, "that which is without limit" or "the Illimitable." According to Chinese philosophy Wu Chi is where all things are produced and T'ai Chi is the product. This term was first introduced by the Taoist, Chou Tun-yi, of the Sung dynasty as a philosophical theory of a mind without thought or desire, hence, a mind without limit.

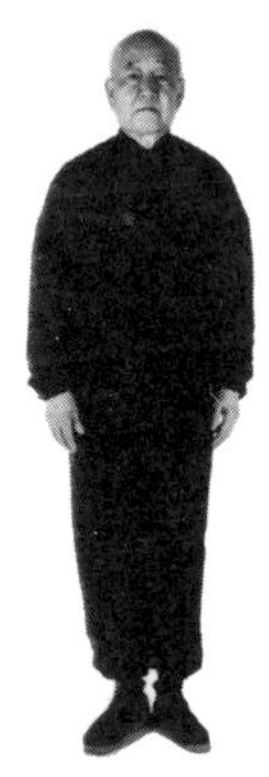

POSTURE 1

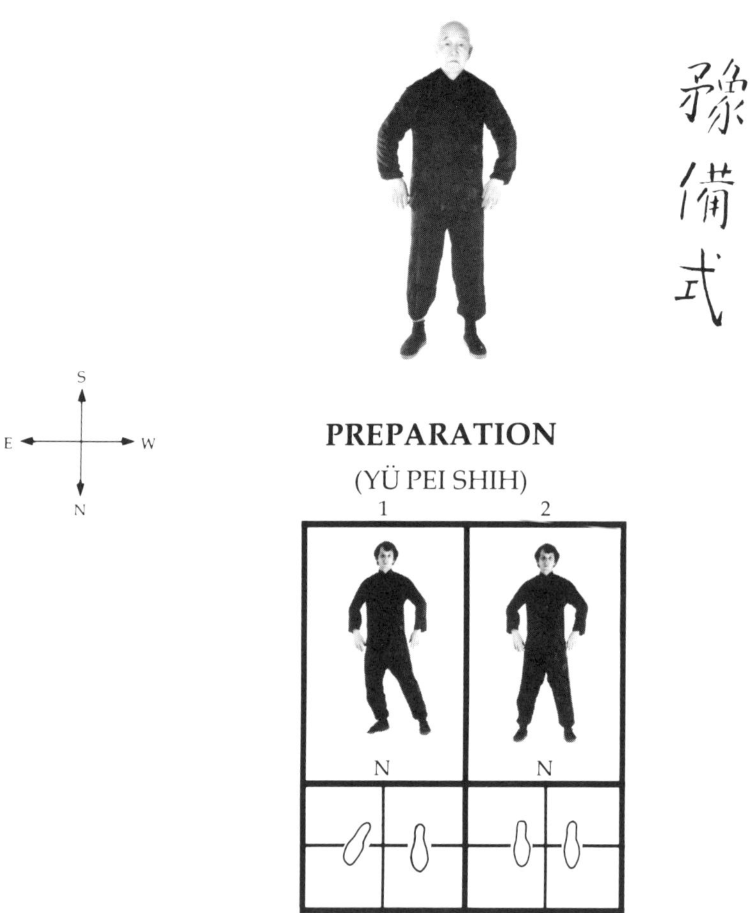

During the Counts of:

1. Shift your weight completely onto the right leg. Raise the left foot and place it sideways about twelve inches to the left, toes pointing directly ahead (north) and rest your weight on it; at the same time bend the elbows slightly outward with the palms facing backward.
2. Pivoting on the right heel, raise the right toes and curve them slightly inward so that the right foot is parallel to the left foot. Both feet are now pointing directly ahead (north). The weight is centered between the two legs; the distance between the feet should be equal to the distance between the shoulders; the shoulders should always be slumped, the chest depressed, with the tongue resting against the hard palate and the mouth lightly closed. The spine should be as straight as possible, the lowest vertebrae hanging in a plumb-line with the head floating as though suspended from above. The entire body should be relaxed completely. It is only then that the **ch'i** can sink to the **tan-tien** (one and one-third inches below the navel).

POSTURE 2

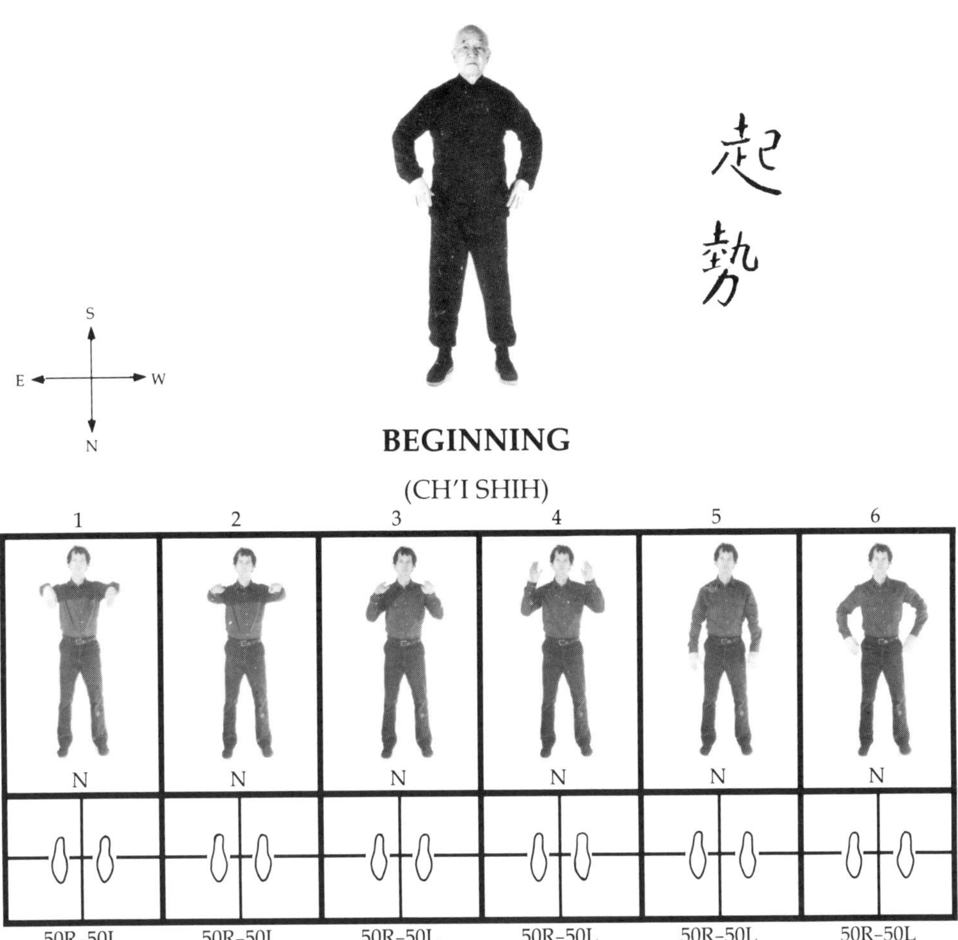

BEGINNING

(CH'I SHIH)

During the Counts of:

1. Looking forward, inhaling slowly, gradually raise the arms forward and upwards to shoulder height with wrists bent, facing up and fingers hanging down.
2. Slowly extend the fingers so that they point forward (north).
3. Bend the elbows slightly and allow the hands to be drawn back towards the upper chest.
4. Lower the elbows slightly downward as the fingers are raised slightly upward.
5. Slowly lower your hands (wrists sinking as though supported by water, fingers floating upward) until they are below the hip joints with palms facing backward.
6. Bend the elbows slightly outward and let the fingers hang downward.

POSTURE 3

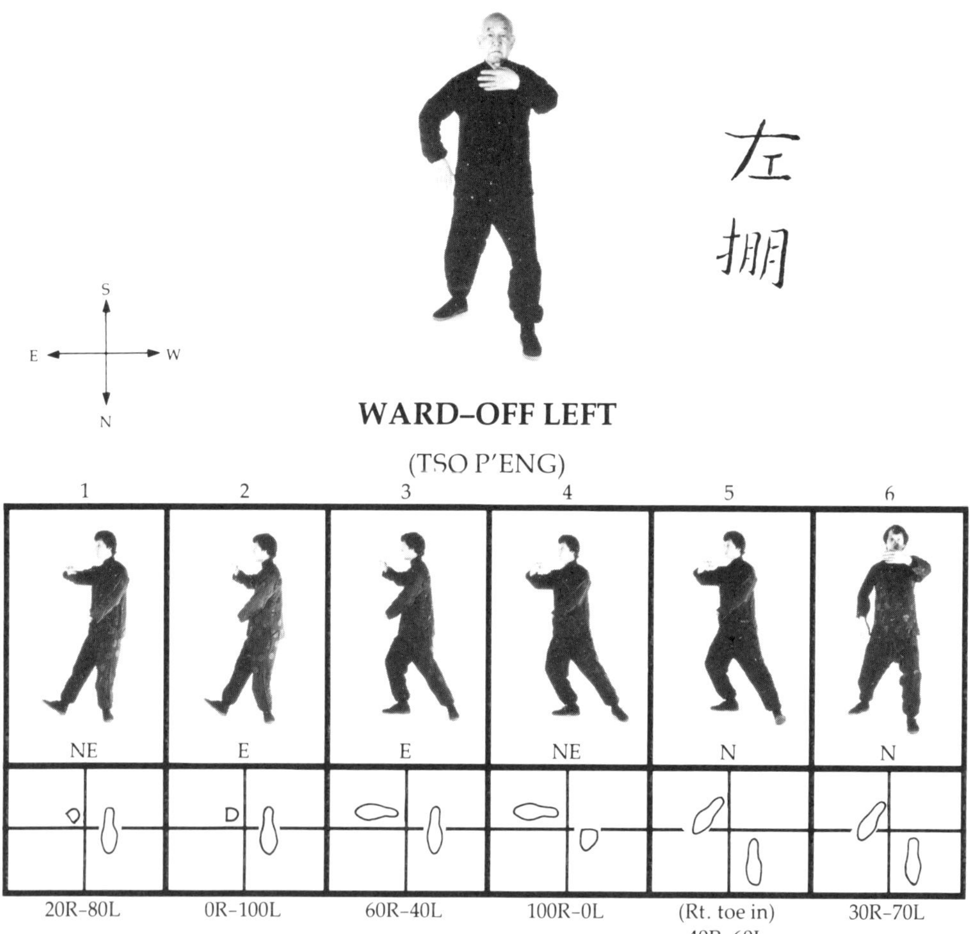

WARD–OFF LEFT

(TSO P'ENG)

During the Counts of:

1. Shift the weight to the left leg and allowing the knees to bend slightly, gradually turn the trunk about 45 degrees to the right (NE).
2. Continue to turn the trunk 45 degrees to the right (east). The toes of the right foot rise up slightly and the foot pivots on the heel to the right (east) so that it is now at a right angle to the left foot. Throughout the turning of the trunk, the legs and arms must be allowed to move simultaneously with the waist and hips. Keep the elbow slightly down while simultaneously raising the right hand gradually, palm down, to the level of the armpit and slowly bring the left hand, palm up, to the level of the right waist. (Note: The arm movement actually begins on Beat #1.) Feel as though a large ball of air were being held between the hands. The eyes have accompanied this movement and are now looking directly ahead (east).
3. Shift the majority of the weight to the right foot.
4. Gradually turn the trunk about 45 degrees to the left (NE) so that the left foot is brought to the tip of the toes.

5. Touching first with the heel, place the left foot directly forward and slowly shift the weight onto it while turning the upper torso to the left. At the same time raise the left arm with the elbow slightly down. Lower the right arm while pivoting on the heel, turning the right foot inward so that the toes point NE. (Note: The picture for this beat does not show it at its completion. It shows the step forward only).
6. Shift 70 percent of your weight to the left foot; simultaneously continue to raise the left arm until the palm of the hand faces your chest and continue to lower the right arm until the hand rests beside the right hip joint, palm backward. The eyes have accompanied this gradual turning movement and now look directly ahead (north).

POSTURE 4

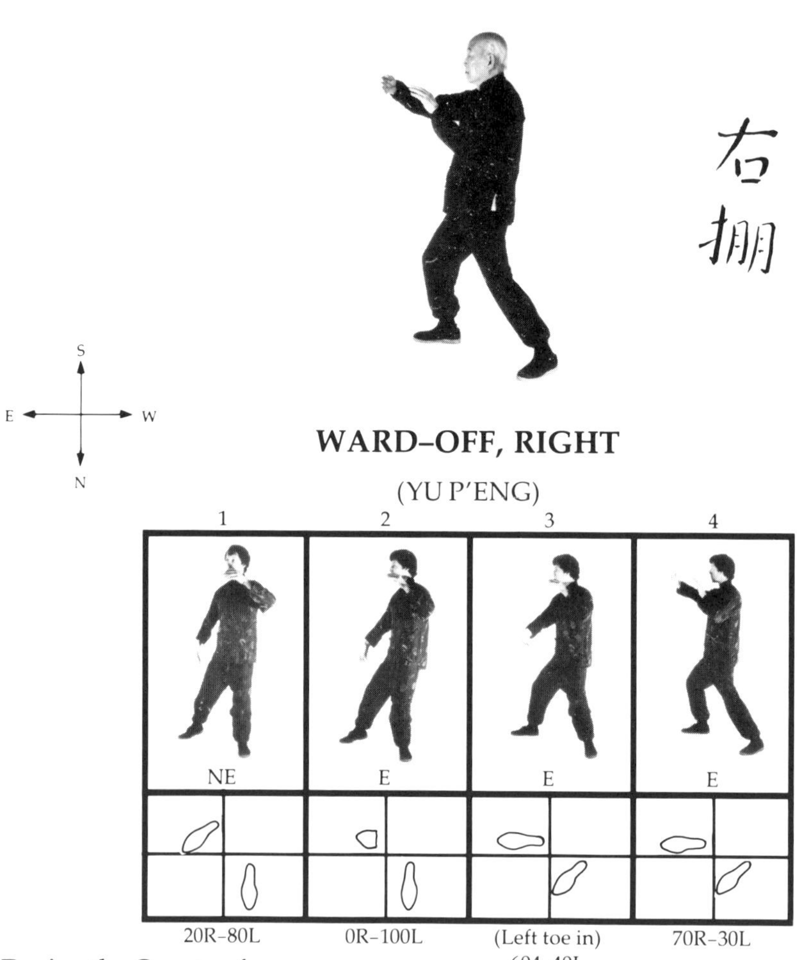

WARD–OFF, RIGHT

(YU P'ENG)

During the Counts of:

1. Shift most of the weight to the left leg and turn the trunk slowly toward the right (NE).
2. Continue to turn the trunk to the right (east) until the right foot is brought to its toe (pointing east); at the same time gradually turn the palms of the hands so that they face each other.
3. Raise the toes off the ground and place the right foot down heel first on the same spot previously occupied by the toes and gradually shift the weight to the foot. At the same time pivot on the left heel and stretching the left leg, slightly turn the left foot inward (NE). (Note: The picture for this beat does not show it at its completion; it does not show the left toe in).
4. Shift 70 percent of the body weight to the bent right leg. At the same time the right arm, with elbow slightly lowered, is carried upwards until the palm faces the upper chest. The left arm, elbow down, moves towards the east until the palm of the hand faces outward with the fingers pointing upwards midway between the upper chest and the right hand. Feel again that a ball of air is being held with the left hand on the near side of the ball and the right hand on the far side of it; the diameter of the ball being about six inches. You are now facing east.

POSTURE 5

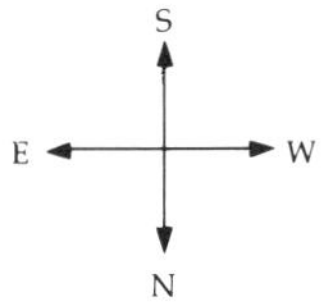

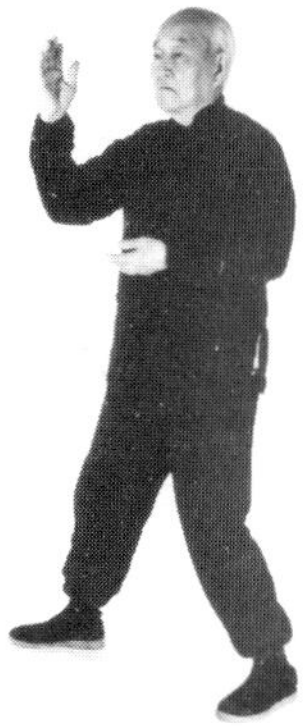

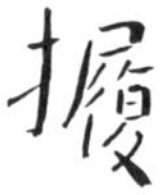

攌

S
E W
N

ROLL BACK

(LÜ)

1	2	3	4
SE	E	E	NE
80R-20L	80R-20L	40R-60L	20R-80L

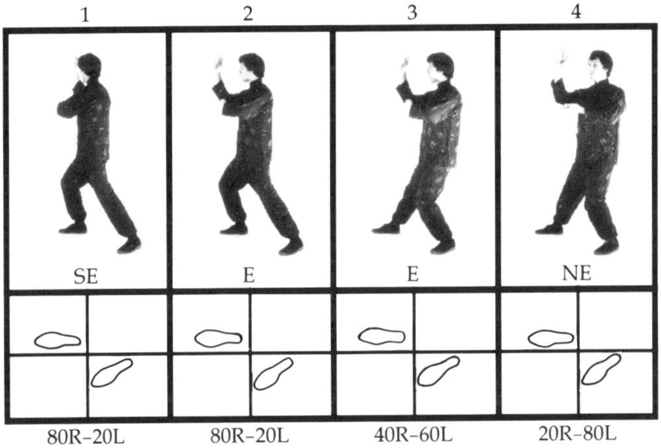

During the Counts of:

1. Gradually turn the torso rightward (to face SE). At the same time extend the right arm slightly, bending the elbow downward so that the fingers point upwards with the palm facing NE. Bend the left elbow slightly downward so that the left hand, palm faces in, is held near the chest at the level of the right elbow (for protection).
2. Gradually turn the torso to the left (to face east). The body and the hands are to act as one unit.
3. Slowly withdraw the weight of the body to the left foot.
4. Bend the left knee to allow the left leg to bear the full weight of the body as the torso turns to the left (NE). At the same time turn your left palm slightly upward in order to disperse your opponent's "push energy." This posture is the epitome of "yield" required in T'ai Chi Ch'uan and it must be done correctly. You are now facing NE.

POSTURE 6

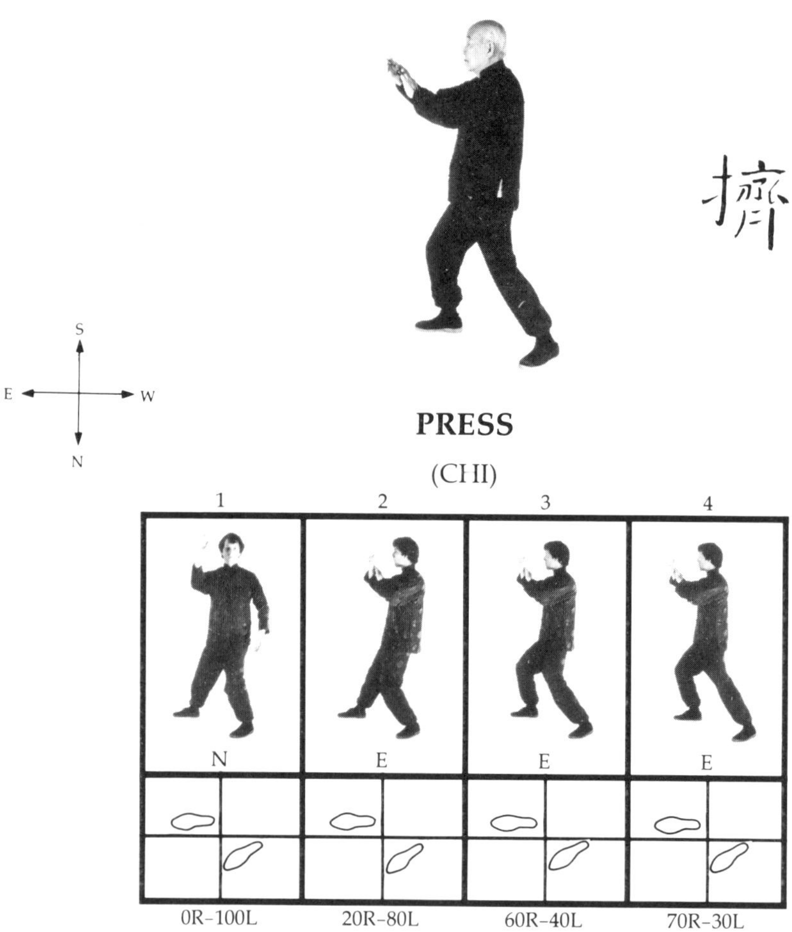

PRESS

(CHI)

During the Counts of:

1. Turn the torso slightly to the left (to face north); let the left hand trace a clockwise circle backward, upward and then forward.
2. Turn the body gradually to the right (east), protecting with the right arm, elbow bent and palm of the hand facing the upper chest. Lightly rest the fingers of the left hand upon the inner wrist of the right hand, for reinforcement.
3. Gradually shift the weight onto the right leg and press forward with the hands together and the body as one unit.
4. Continue to press forward with the hands and body as one unit until the right leg bears 70 percent of the weight. Thus the hands are advanced forward (east) by the body until at the last moment when there is a subtle diagonal upward press (uproot technique to be directed by the mind). You are now facing east.

POSTURE 7

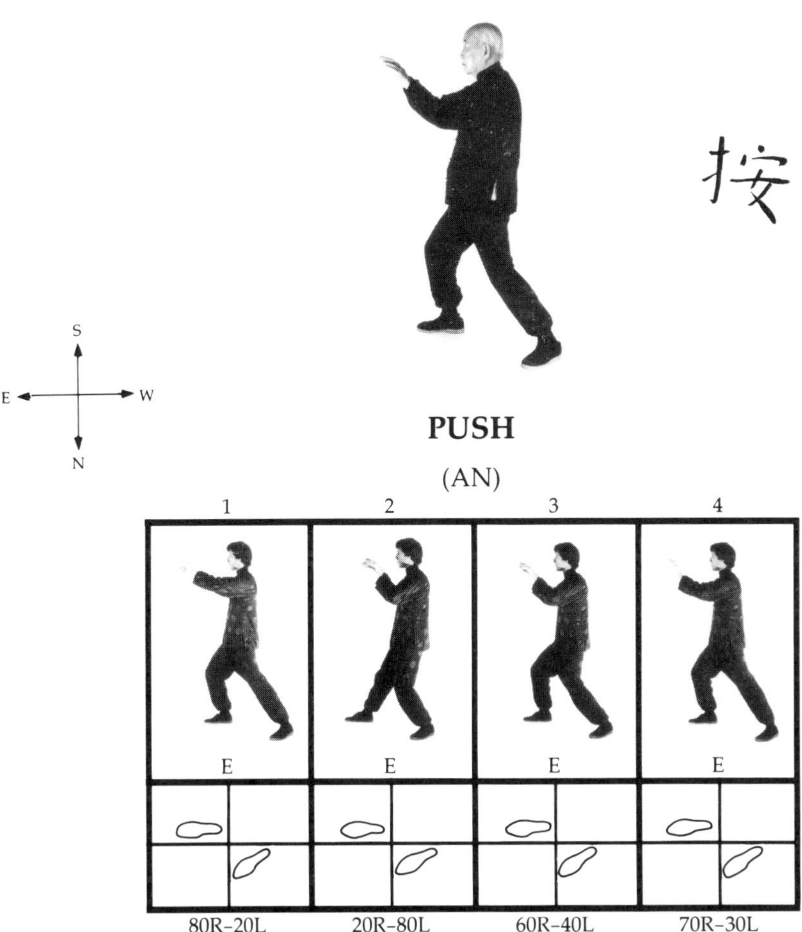

PUSH

(AN)

During the Counts of:

1. Separate your hands, palms down, at the level of your shoulders with arms slightly stretched and begin to withdraw your body backwards.
2. Continue to withdraw your body backward until the weight of the entire body is shifted onto the left leg. As the arms are withdrawn, the elbows hang down and the palms of the hands face outward with the wrists at the level of the shoulders.
3. With the whole body rooted and moving as one unit, begin to push forward (the arms are an integral part of the forward intention).
4. Continue to push forward until 70 percent of your weight has been shifted to your right leg and the last moment perform a subtle diagonal upward push (uproot technique). (The elbows are still bent: the palms are outward: the wrists are not bent and do not break the smooth line from elbows to finger tips). Arm movements must issue from the trunk; if the arms act independently the exercise is worthless. This rule applies to every posture. Heed it well. You are still facing east.

POSTURE 8

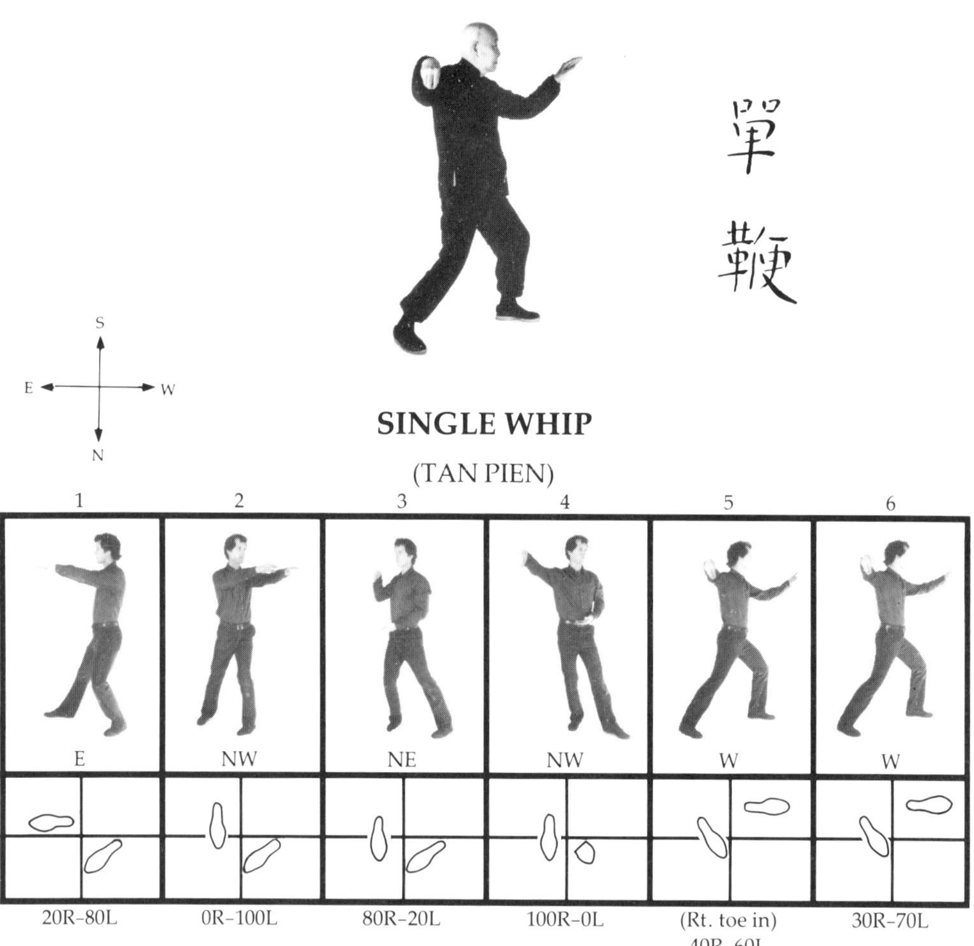

During the Counts of:

1. Shift your weight gradually to the left foot with the palms of the hands facing downward and hands parallel with the shoulders.
2. Turn your torso to the left until it faces northwest and at the same time swivel on the right heel, curving the toes inward as far as possible.
3. As the weight is shifted back to the right leg, allow the body to turn to the right (so that it will be facing NE) and as the elbow bends withdraw the right arm. Allow the fingers to point downward and close together at the fingertips, thus forming a ''hook'' near the right armpit. Bring the left hand to rest, palm up, near the right breast.
4. As the torso turns gradually leftward (to face the northwest corner) and swivels on the ball of the left foot so that the toes point northwest extend the ''hook'' hand rightward so that the knuckles face the northwest corner.
5. As the trunk continues to turn leftward, take a wide step to the SW with the left foot. First set the heel down, then toes to point west; shift the weight to the leg. The left heel should not be directly in front of the right heel but on as

wide a diagonal position as can be comfortably managed. At the same time turn the right foot inward maintaining contact on the floor with the heel. The left hand, palm turning inward, is carried leftward until it is opposite the left breast. Throughout this movement the eyes gaze at the palm of the hand.

6. Gradually shift 70% of the body weight to the left leg, bending the leg at the knee, and allow your waist to turn leftward so that it faces west. At the same time turn the left hand palm outward with the arm slightly bent, as the eyes, which have accompanied the gradual turn, look past the fingertips. You are now facing west.

POSTURE 9

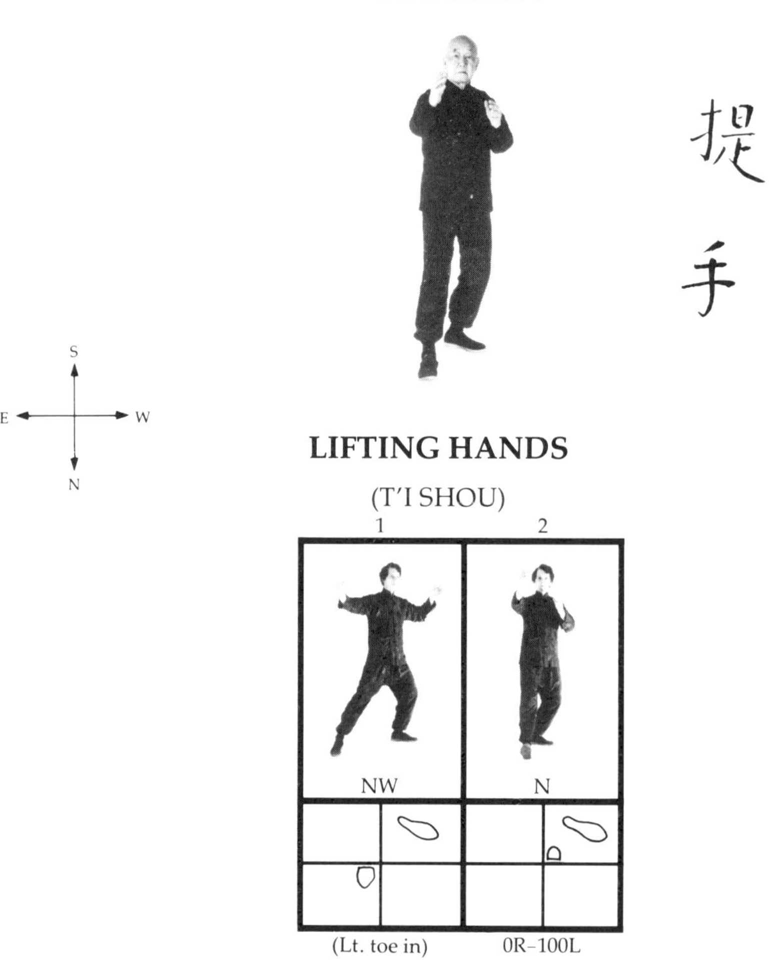

LIFTING HANDS

(T'I SHOU)

During the Counts of:

1. Shift the weight onto the right leg and turn in the left foot slightly. Then as you turn your torso rightward (to face north), shift all your weight back to your left leg, allowing the right heel to raise. Turn your palms inward so that they face each other.
2. Carry your right foot leftward until you can place the heel (toes pointing up) on the ground about a foot's length in front of your left heel. At the same time slowly bring your arms toward each other so that your right elbow is slightly bent and aligned over your right leg in advance of your left arm. Your left arm, elbow slightly bent, has the palms facing (about 12″ apart) the crook of the right elbow. The hands and the legs must move and stop at the same time. As it says in the T'ai Chi Ch'uan classics, ''When you act, everything moves and when you stand still, everything is tranquil.'' You are now facing north.

POSTURE 10

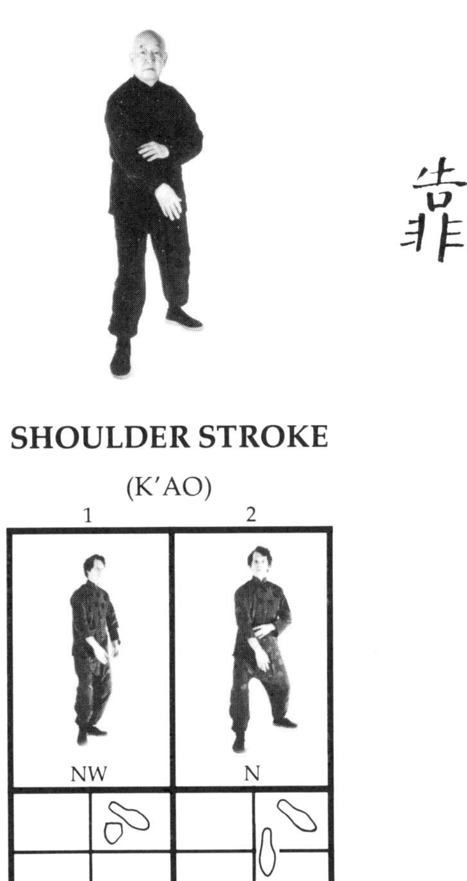

SHOULDER STROKE

(K'AO)

During the Counts of:

1. Bring your right foot back and place it down on the ball of the foot with the toes directly in front (north) of your left heel. At the same time retract and lower your right hand and let it hang, palm inward so that the outer edge of the hand is near the front of your right thigh. Lower your left hand and let it hang, palm outward, so that its outer edge is near the outer left thigh.
2. Step forward with your right foot (heel touching first) and shift 70% of your weight to it. Lightly apply your left hand to the crook of your right forearm for reinforcement. Using the tenacious energy of your left foot strike forward (north) with your right shoulder.

POSTURE 11

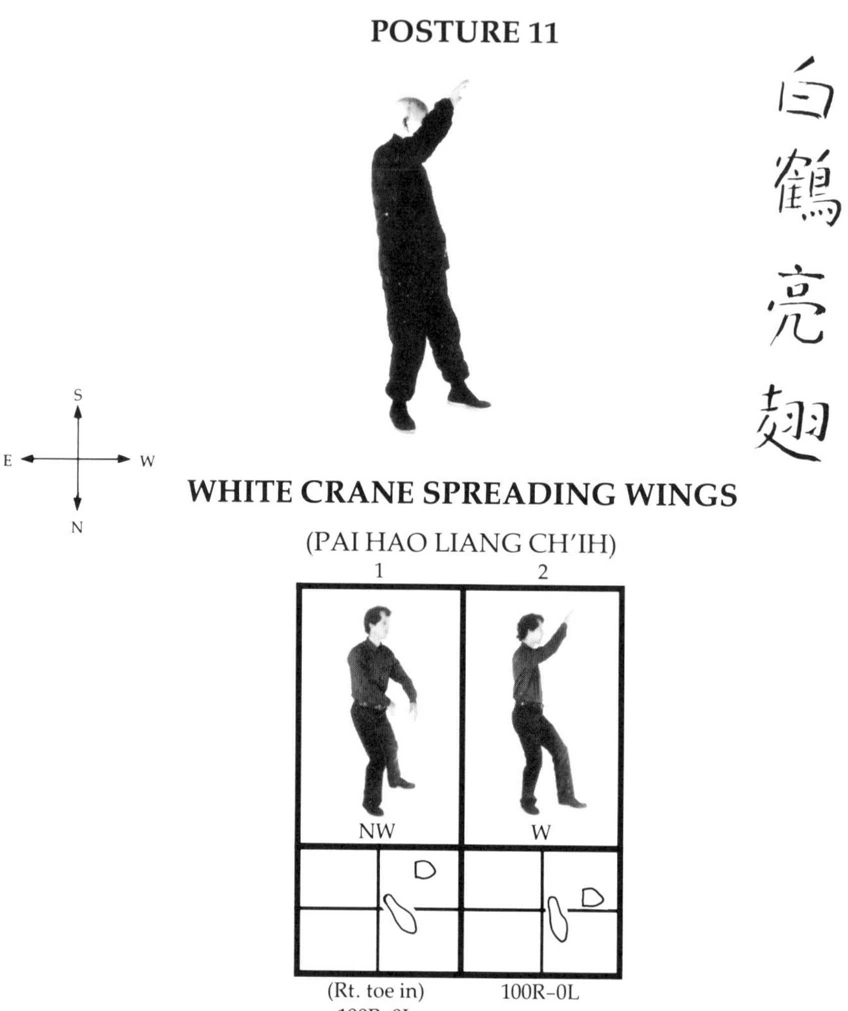

WHITE CRANE SPREADING WINGS

(PAI HAO LIANG CH'IH)

During the Counts of:

1. Shift your weight back to the left foot and turn your right foot slightly inward. Shift all your weight to your right foot as you turn leftward (to face west), allowing the left heel to rise slightly (the ball and toes remaining on the ground, pointing west). Begin to raise your right arm, tracing about 90 degrees of a large clockwise circle, and begin to lower your left arm.
2. Bring your left foot forward (along a diagonally right line) and place only its toes down so that they are in alignment with your right heel (about 8″ in front of it). At the same time raise your right arm through another 90 degree circle until your right elbow hangs at the level of your chin and your right hand (palm forward, fingers pointing upward) is above your head. Continue to lower your left arm until the hand rests beside your left hip joint, its palm facing backward. You are now facing west.

POSTURE 12

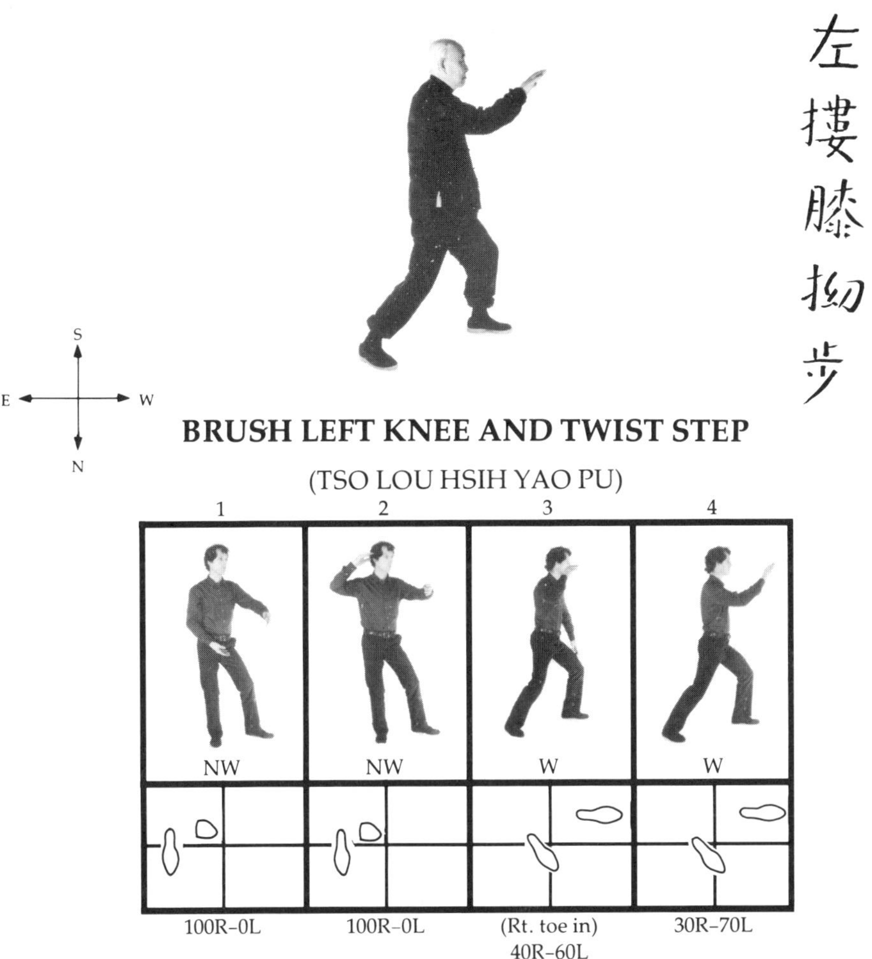

左摟膝拗步

BRUSH LEFT KNEE AND TWIST STEP

(TSO LOU HSIH YAO PU)

During the Counts of:

1. Lower the body on a slightly bended right knee and turn the torso slightly to the right. At the same time your right hand, palm up, is to be turned and lowered beside the right thigh; begin circling the left hand to the right clockwise, until the palm is facing you. (Note: Although the direction indicated is northwest the trunk has not reached this position until beat #2).
2. Continue to turn the trunk to the right facing northwest, and with the right hand circle in a counter-clockwise path: backward, upward and forward until the palm comes beside the right ear, facing forward (west), elbow bent. Continue circling the left hand until it faces the right side of the chest with the fingers pointing north.
3. Gradually turn the body to the left (west). Take a step diagonally forward (left) with the left foot, heel touching the ground first, and brush the left knee with the left hand, palm facing backwards; let it rest (stop) beside the left thigh. Bring the right arm, elbow bent, in front of the chest. At the same time

gradually shift the weight to the left foot and rotating on the right heel, turn your right foot slightly inward.

4. Gradually shift 70% of the body weight to the left foot and using the intrinsic energy of the entire body, push forward with the right hand, elbow slightly bent. You are still facing west.

POSTURE 13

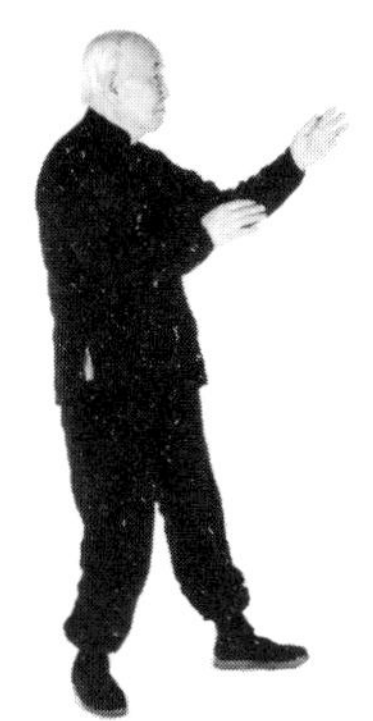

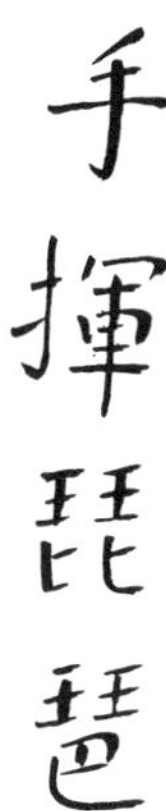

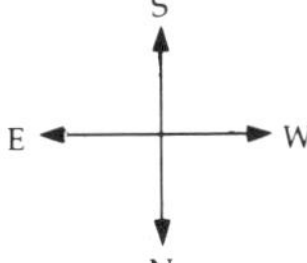

PLAYING THE GUITAR

(SHOU HUI P'I PA)

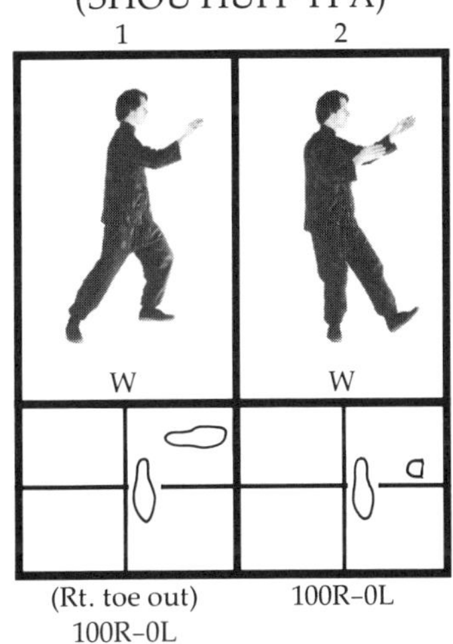

During the Counts of:

1. Pick up your right foot, turn it 30 degrees to the right, set it down and shift the entire body weight to it. (Note: The picture for this beat does not show it at its completion; it shows the right toe out only).
2. Shift your left foot slightly sideways to the right and touch the ground with the heel only, which should be in line with the right heel. At the same time bring the right hand along in a backward arc, palm facing south, and carry it to a position opposite the left elbow, raising the left hand, palm facing north, so that the fingers are in line with the mouth. The elbow is slightly bent and the fingers point west. The position simulates playing a guitar. You are still facing west.

POSTURE 14

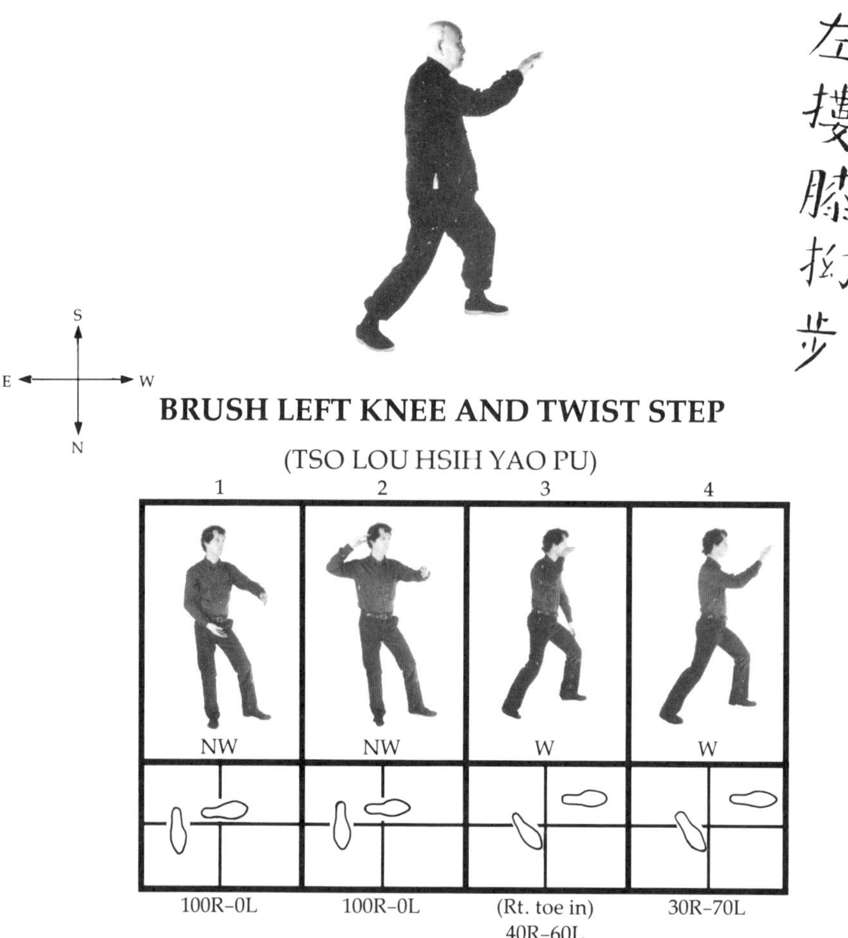

BRUSH LEFT KNEE AND TWIST STEP

(TSO LOU HSIH YAO PU)

During the Counts of:

1. This beat is the same as posture #12, beat 1, except that the left foot drops but no weight is placed on it. Beats 2, 3, and 4 are the same as the respective beats of posture #12.

POSTURE 15

右摟膝拗步

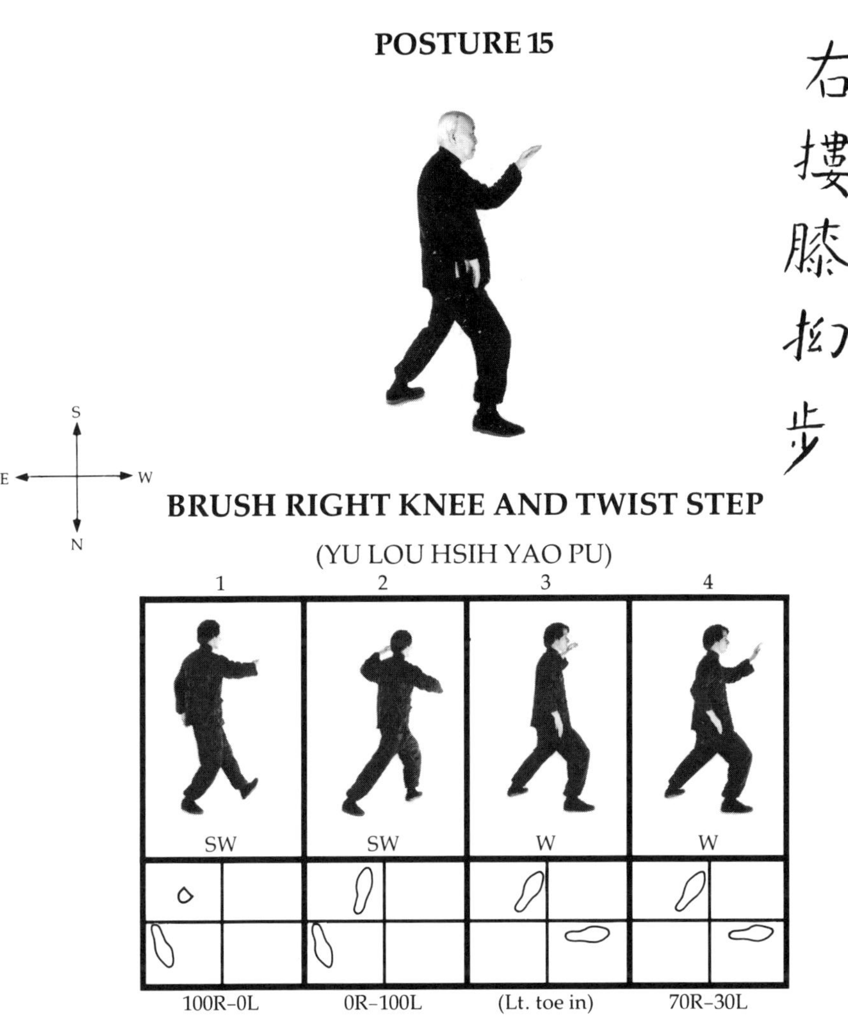

BRUSH RIGHT KNEE AND TWIST STEP

(YU LOU HSIH YAO PU)

During the Counts of:

1. Withdraw the body weight to the right foot and turn the torso slightly to the left, curving the left toes slightly outward to point southwest. At the same time draw the right hand down and leftward until the palm faces the chest and turn the left hand outward facing west.
2. Shift the body weight to the left foot and circle the left hand clockwise, backward, upward, and forward to the left ear. This palm should be facing outward and slightly inclined downward with this elbow bent.
3. Turn the torso slightly to the right and take a big step forward with the right foot, heel touching the ground first. Brush the right knee with the right hand, palm backward, bringing it to rest beside the right thigh. Begin shifting the body weight to the right foot and curve the left foot slightly inward, turning on the heel.
4. When 70% of the body weight is on the right foot, with the intrinsic energy of your entire body push the left hand forward, with the elbow slightly bent. You are still facing west.

POSTURE 16

BRUSH LEFT KNEE AND TWIST STEP

(TSO LOU HSIH YAO PU)

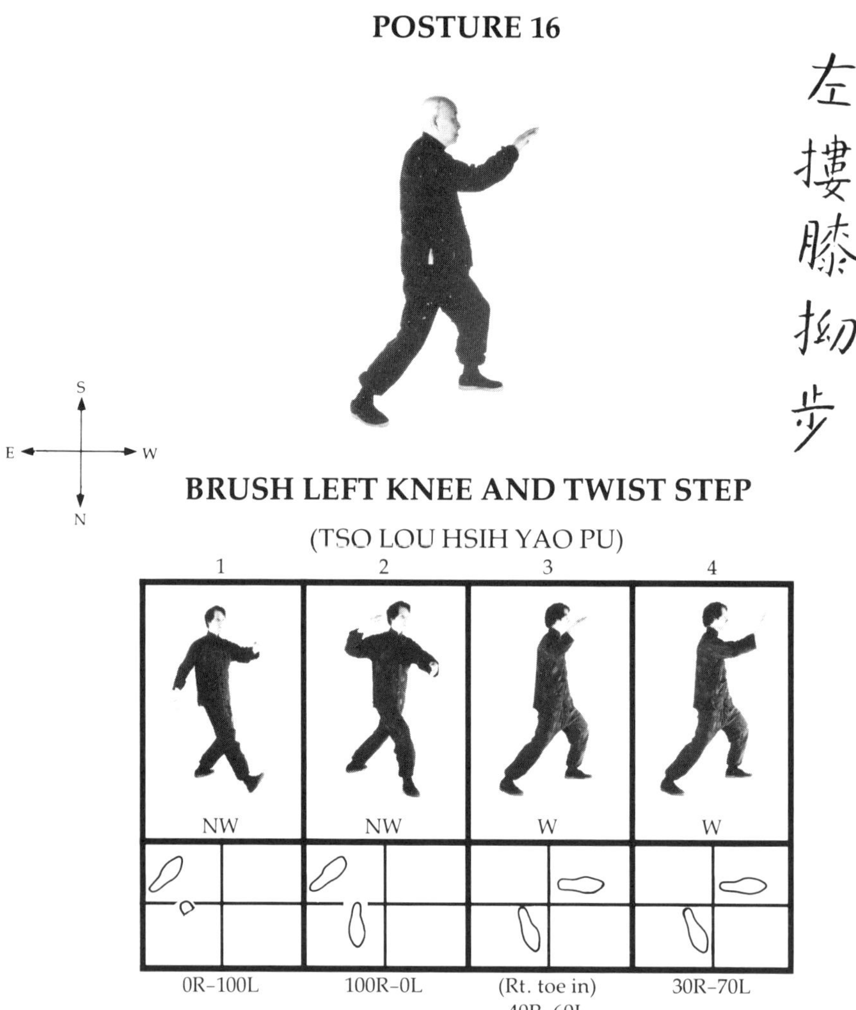

During the Counts of:

1. As the body weight is withdrawn onto the left foot, turn the torso slightly to the right and turn the right foot slightly outward so that it points northwest. At the same time turn the right hand so that the palm faces west and draw the left hand down so that the palm faces your right chest area.
2. Shift the body weight to the right foot and circle the right hand counter-clockwise from downward to upward until it is by the right ear, palm facing forward and slightly inclined, with the elbow bent downward.

Beats 3 and 4 are the same as the respective beats of posture #12.

POSTURE 17

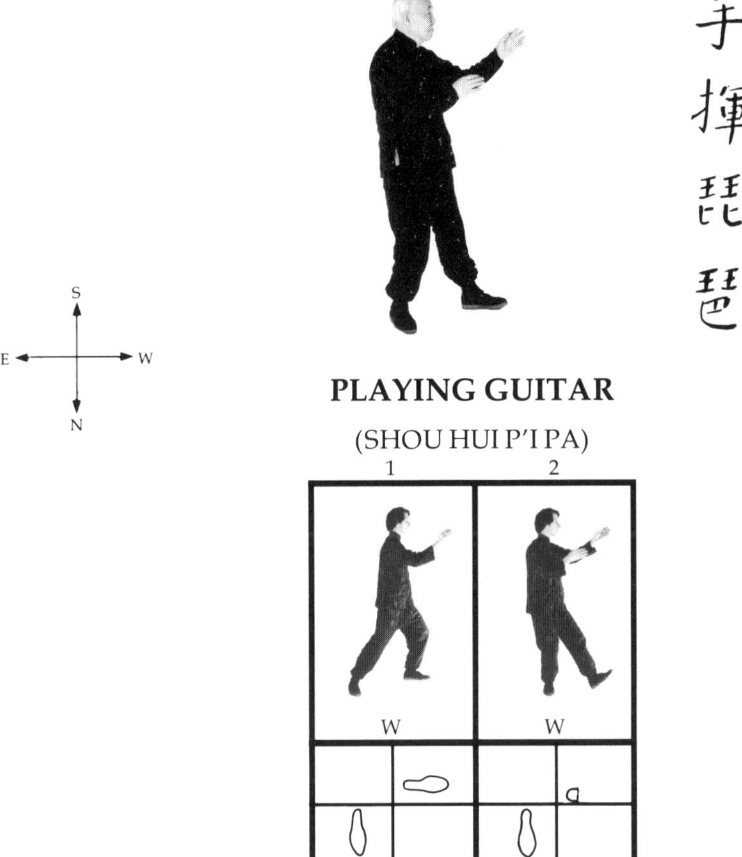

PLAYING GUITAR

(SHOU HUI P'I PA)

This posture is the same as posture #13.

POSTURE 18

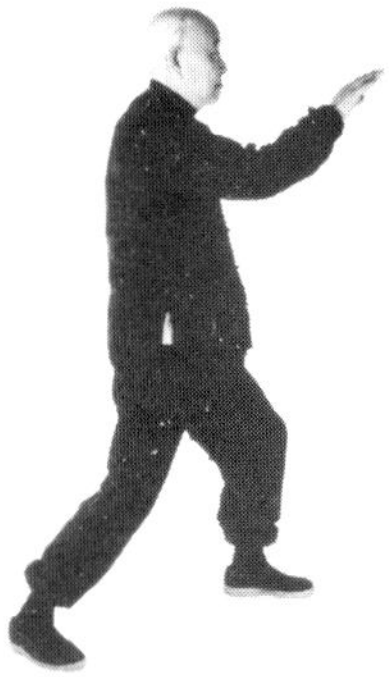

左摟膝拗步

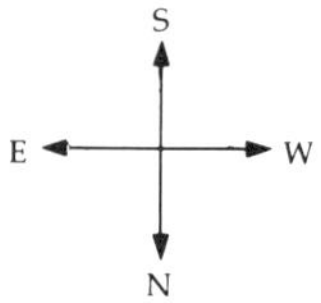

S
E W
N

BRUSH LEFT KNEE AND TWIST STEP

(TSO LOU HSIH YAO PU)

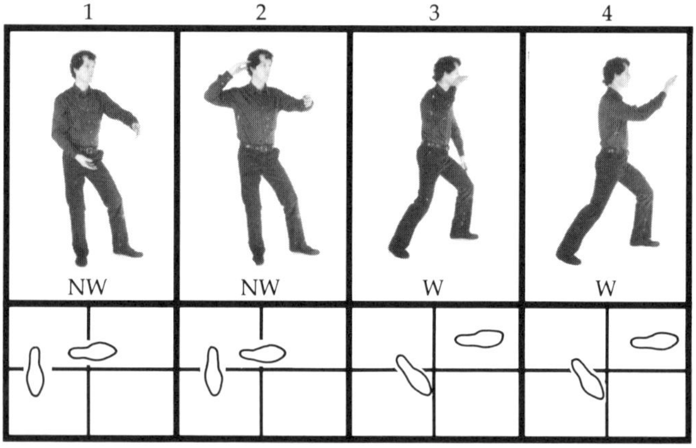

1	2	3	4
NW	NW	W	W

This beat is the same as posture #12, beat 1, except that the left foot drops but no weight is placed on it.
Beats 2, 3, and 4 are the same as the respective beats of posture #12.

POSTURE 19

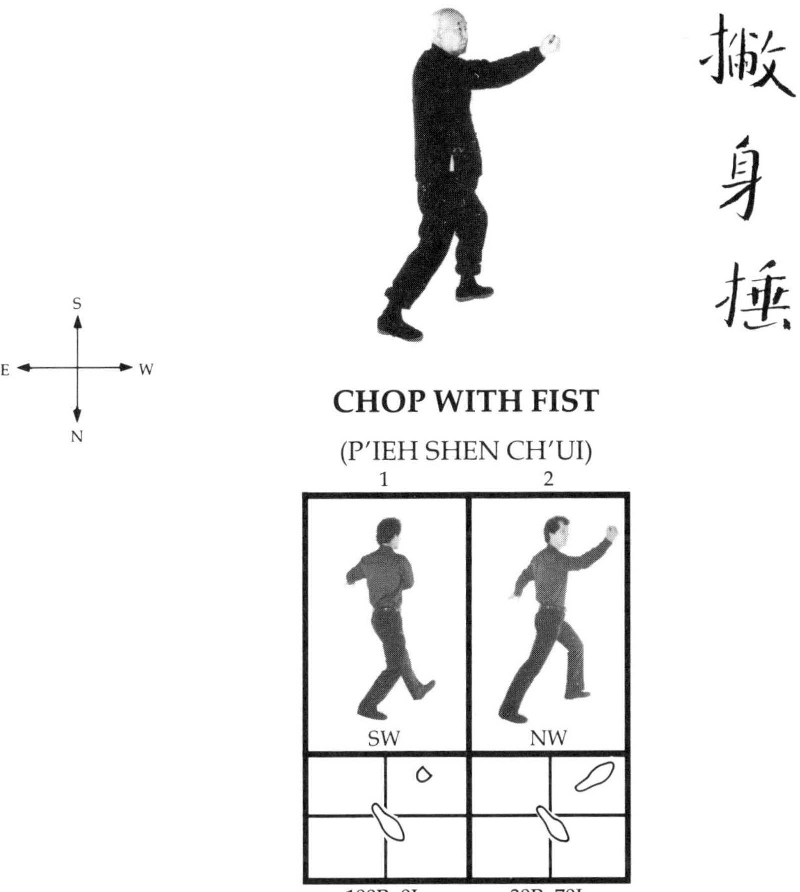

撇身捶

CHOP WITH FIST

(P'IEH SHEN CH'UI)

During the Counts of:

1. Draw the body back to shift the weight to your right foot and pivot on your left heel to turn the raised foot slightly outward, pointing southwest; lower the right hand leftward until the palm faces the left thigh.
2. Shift 70% of the body weight to the left foot; turn the body slightly to the right (NW) and at the same time clench your right hand into a fist and chop upward in a forward direction toward the northwest. The knuckles are downward at the height of your nose. Raise your left hand backward until it rests at the height of the waist, palm down. You are now facing northwest and looking at your right fist.

POSTURE 20

進步搬攔捶

STEP FORWARD, DEFLECT DOWNWARD INTERCEPT AND PUNCH

(CHIN PU PAN LAN CH'UI)

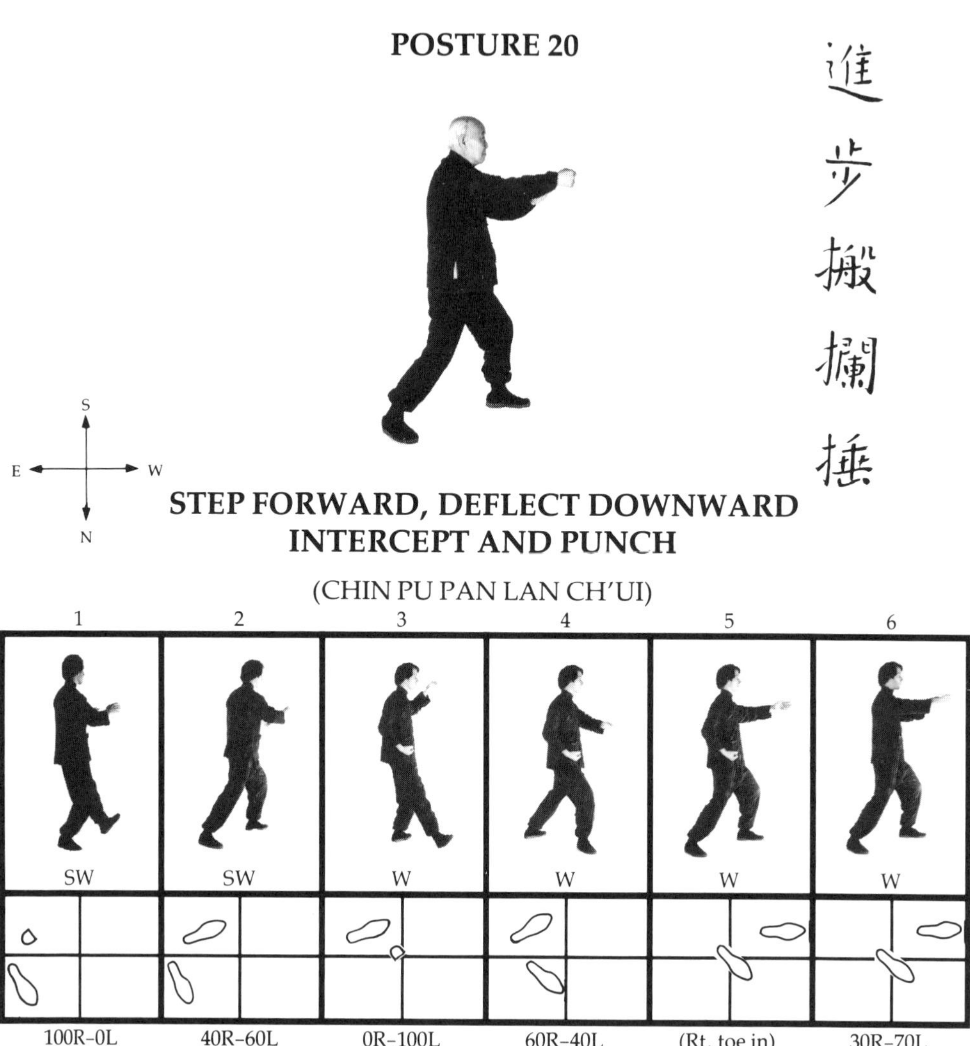

During the Counts of:

1. Withdraw the weight of your right foot, turn the torso slightly to the left, facing southwest and raise the left toes. At the same time open the right fist, turn the hand palm down, and lower it near your left waist; lower the left hand, palm up, close to the left hip joint.
2. Shift the weight to the left foot.
3. Raise the right foot and take a short step diagonally to the forward right direction with only the heel touching the ground. At the same time make a fist with the right hand, with knuckles down, and bring it back to rest under the right side of the waist (deflect); raise the left hand and circle it clockwise, backward, upward and forward near the left ear with the elbow bent and palm facing west.
4. As you sink the body downward, shift the weight to your right foot and let the left hand move forward and downward to be held in front of your right chest with palm down, for protection and interception.

5. Step forward with the left foot and gradually shift 60% of the weight to it; extend the left hand forward and leftward, fingers pointing west and the palm facing north. Curve your right foot slightly inward. Draw the right fist back alongside the right hip, with palm facing up.
6. Shift 70% of the body weight to the left foot and punch forward with the right fist, with tiger's mouth upward (''tiger's mouth'' is the space between the crook of the index finger and thumb). Draw back the left hand so that it slides past the advancing right fist and comes to rest on the inside of the inner wrist of the right hand. You are now facing west.

POSTURE 21

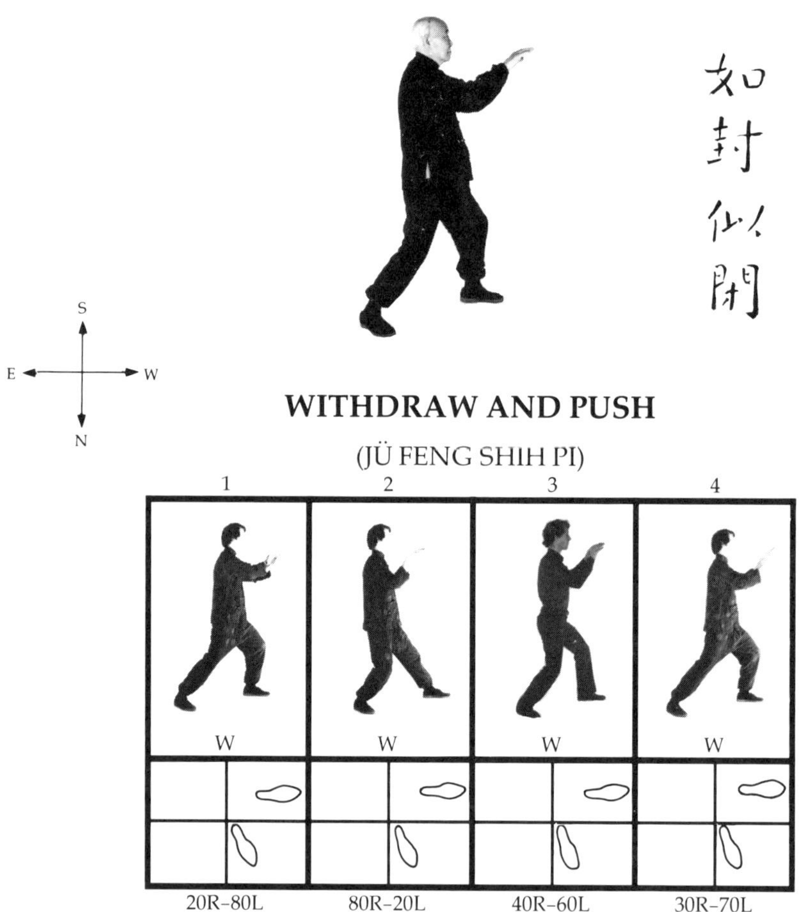

WITHDRAW AND PUSH

(JÜ FENG SHIH PI)

During the Counts of:

1. Gradually withdraw the body, shifting the weight to the right foot, and open the right fist so that the palm is upward. Turn the left palm upward and slide it under the right hand.
2. Continue to shift the weight back until all of it is on the right foot; draw both hands back close to the shoulders with palms facing your chest, and separate the hands turning the palms outward with elbows bent.
3. Begin to push forward by shifting the weight 60% on to the left foot.
4. Continue to push forward with palms outward and arms slightly bent until 70% of the body weight is shifted to the left foot. You are still facing west.

POSTURE 22

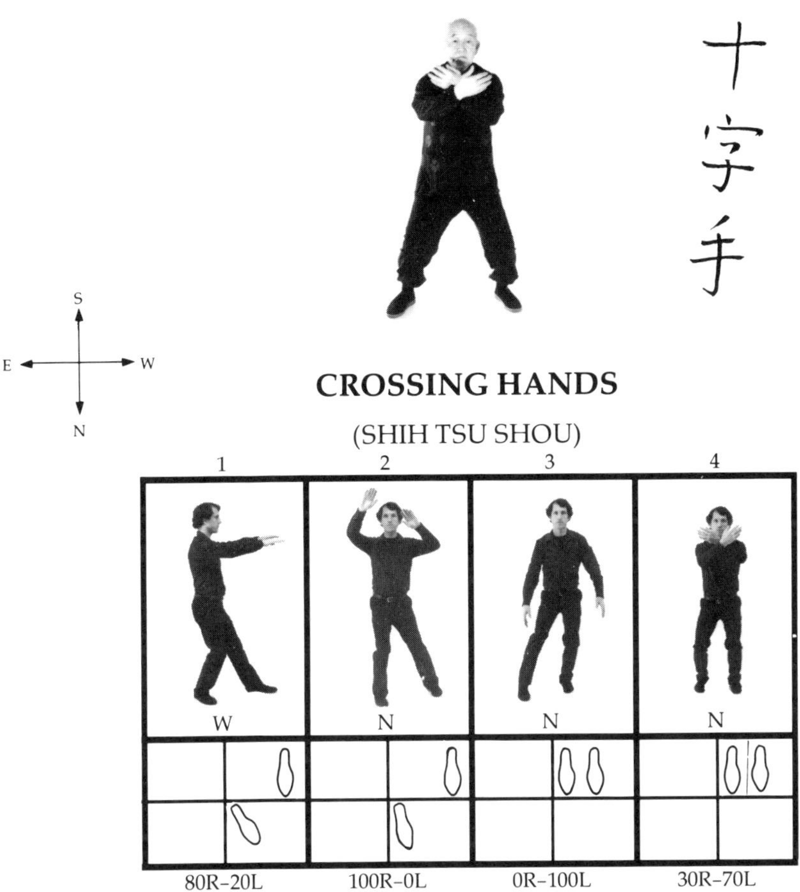

CROSSING HANDS

(SHIH TSU SHOU)

During the Counts of:

1. Gradually shift the body weight onto the right leg and slightly stretch the arms forward with palms downward.
2. Begin turning the body to the right (north), pivoting on the left heel until the foot moving inward points north. Let the right hand be carried along the upward arc of a high circle, with the left hand guided by the turning waist, following the right hand along the same trajectory.
3. As all the body weight is shifted to the left foot, pivot on the right toes to turn the right heel inward and gradually lower both hands in opposite directions and down the sides of the circle (right hand, clockwise), (left hand, counter-clockwise).
4. Bring the right foot back and place it parallel to the left foot, shoulder width apart, so that both feet point directly ahead (north); the knees are slightly bent and the weight of the body is mostly on the left foot.

As the hands approach each other along the lower arc of the circle, cross them diagonally at the wrists and bring them up in front of the chest, palms facing you with the right wrist outside the left wrist. You are now facing north.

POSTURE 23

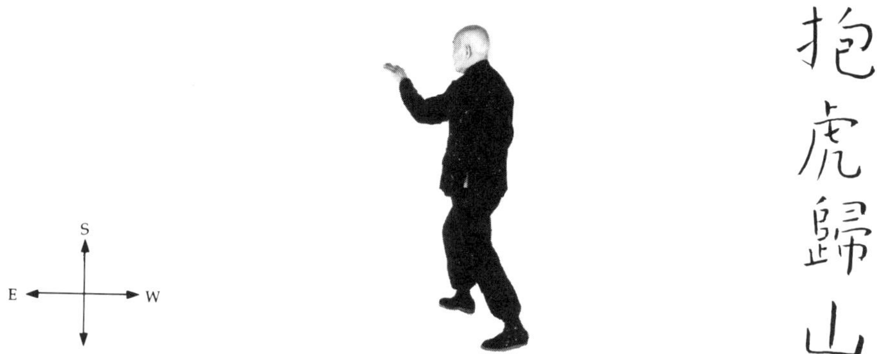

EMBRACE THE TIGER TO RETURN TO THE MOUNTAIN

(PAO HU KUEI SHAN)

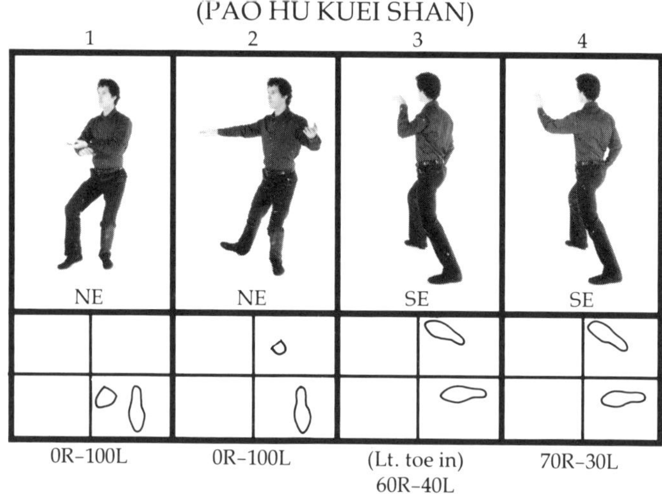

During the Counts of:

1. Gradually turn your body to the right (NE) and turn your right palm down and your left palm up. At the same time turn your right heel slightly leftward with toes touching the ground.
2. Continue to turn your body to the right and take a step with your right foot to the far right (SE) with the heel touching first. At the same time lower both hands and together with the right foot move the right hand towards the southeast with the palm downward, and circle the left hand clockwise in a backwards direction.
3. Continue to move your right hand rightward and backward and place it beside your right thigh with palm upward. The left hand makes a clockwise circle downward, backward and upward; it stops past the left ear with palm forward and elbow bent. Turn your left foot slightly inward, pivoting on the heel and shift 60% of the weight to the right foot.
4. Shift 70% of your weight to the right foot. With the intrinsic energy of your whole body, push your left hand forward (SE) without bending the wrist and the fingers diagonally upward. You are now facing southeast.

POSTURE 24

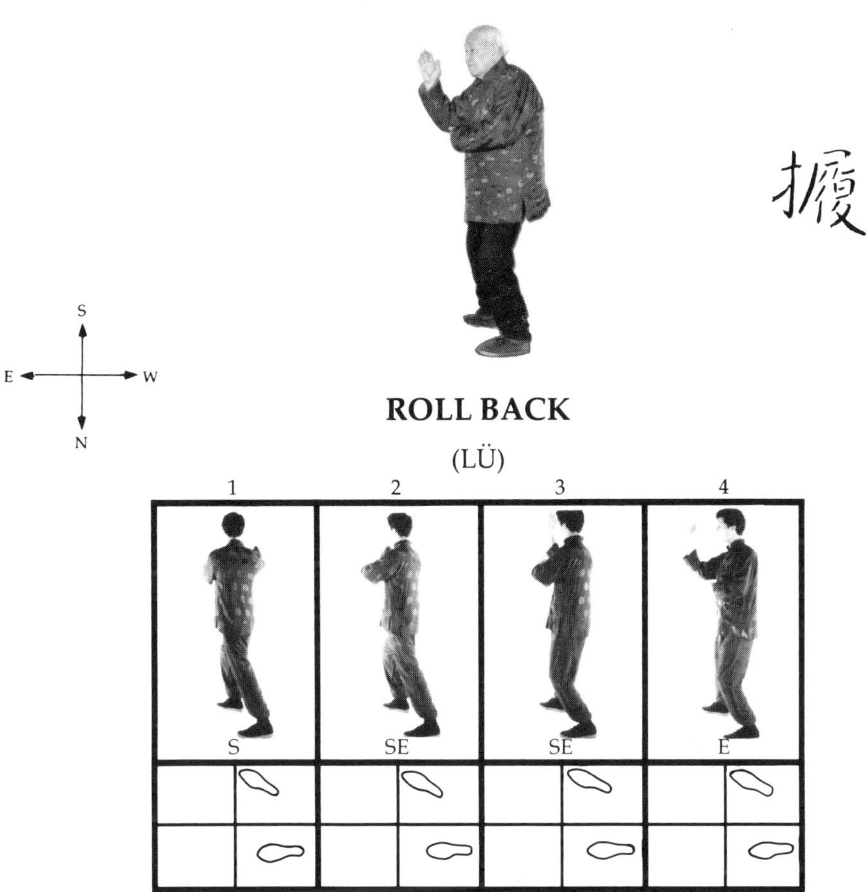

ROLL BACK

(LÜ)

This posture is the same as posture #5.

POSTURE 25

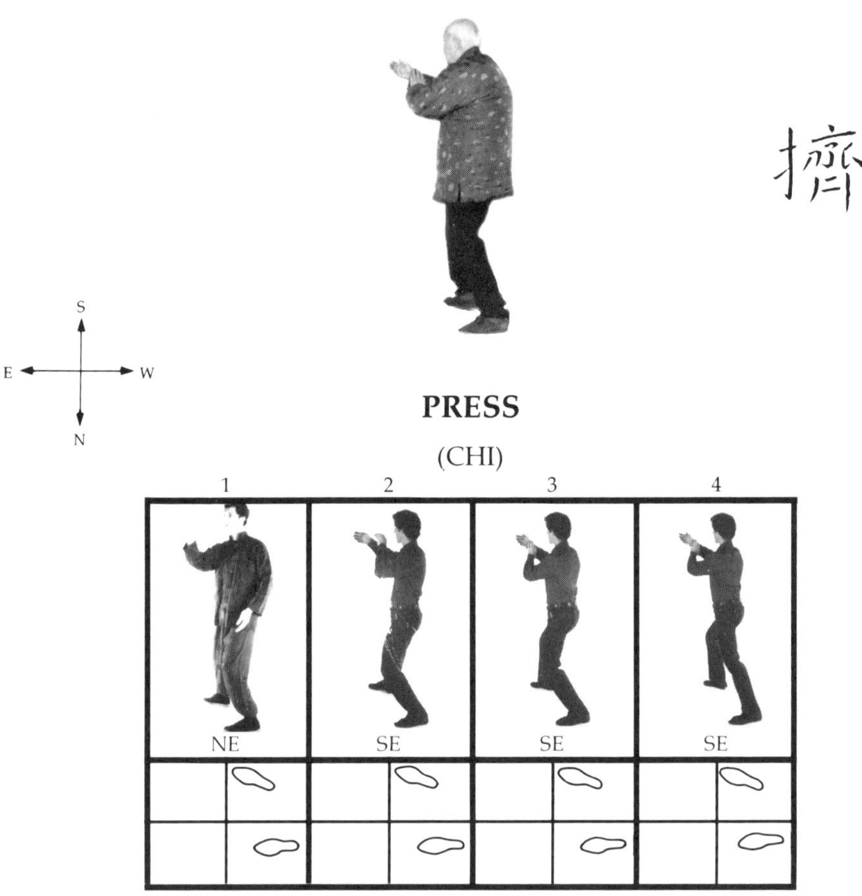

PRESS

(CHI)

This posture is the same as posture #6.

POSTURE 26

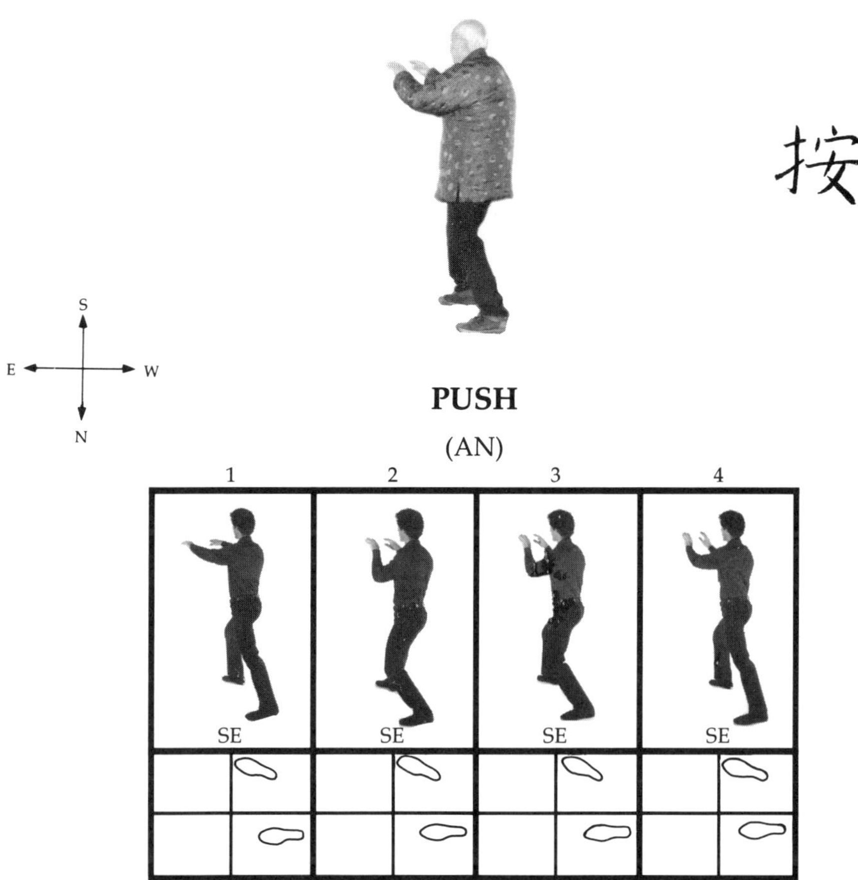

PUSH

(AN)

This posture is the same as posture #7.

POSTURE 27

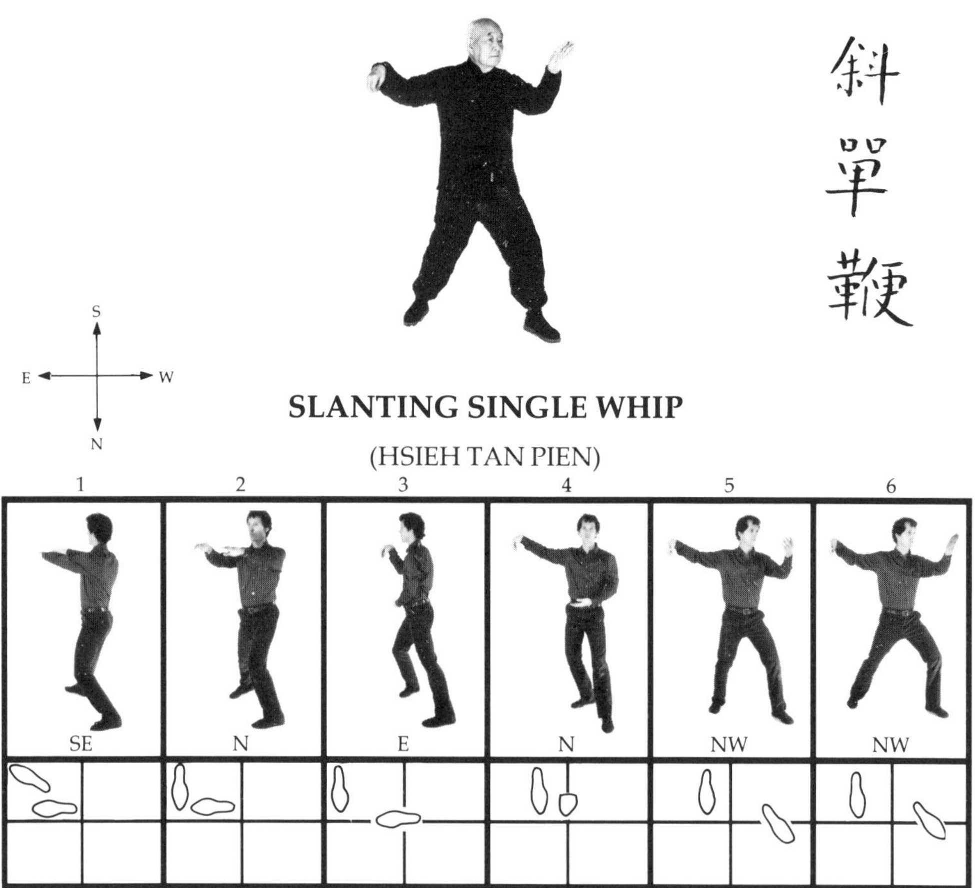

SLANTING SINGLE WHIP

(HSIEH TAN PIEN)

This posture is the same as posture #8.

POSTURE 28

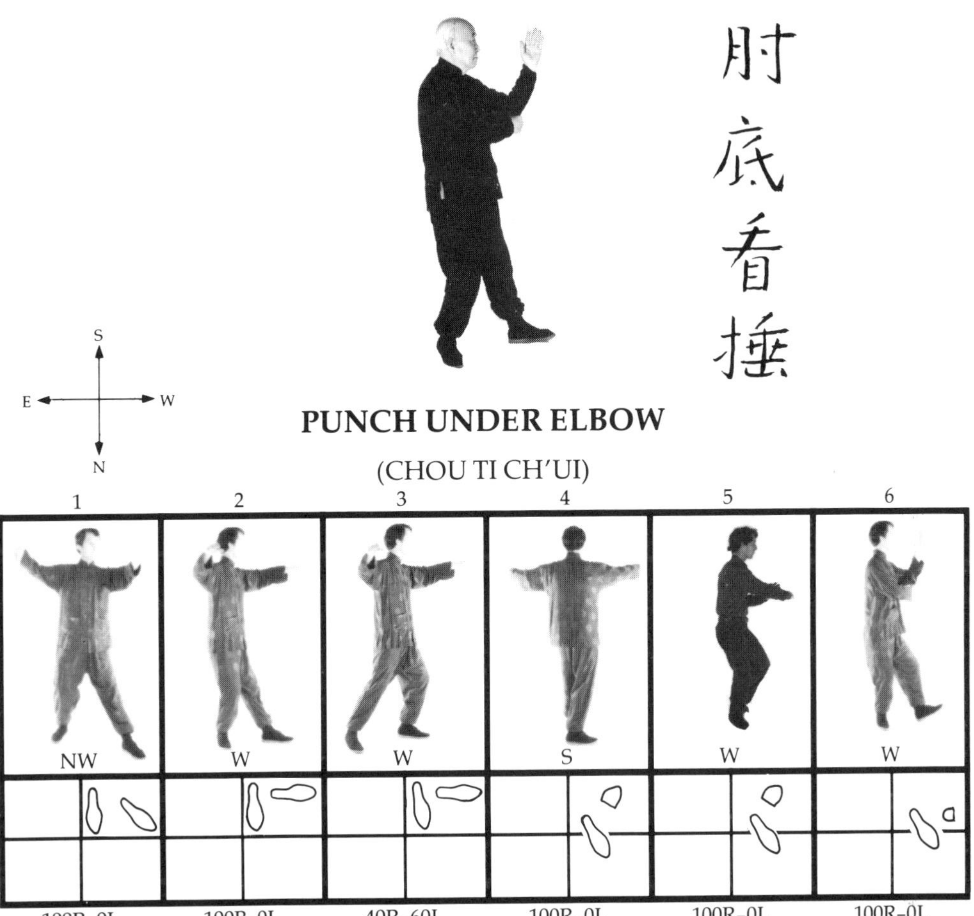

PUNCH UNDER ELBOW

(CHOU TI CH'UI)

During the Counts of:

1. Shift your weight back to your right leg.
2. Turn your body to the left and take one step to the left with your left foot, with toes pointing west. At the same time open the right hand "hook".
3. Shift the weight to the left foot.
4. Bring your right foot to the forward right direction on a line north of your left heel and with the toes pointing northwest. Shift your weight to your right leg, immediately turn your upper torso further to the left (south) with your arms evenly extended on either side, with palms downward.
5. When you have turned your upper torso as far as you can (facing south) and your right hand (extended toward the west) is opposite your left shoulder, start to lower your left hand and circle it downward to the right and upward from beneath your left armpit. At the same time turn your upper torso to the right.
6. Continue to circle your left hand up and inside the right forearm until the fingers are pointing almost vertically upward. At the same time take a one-

half step with your left foot diagonally to the front center, with only the heel touching and in line with your right heel. Make a fist with your right hand (''tiger's mouth'' facing up) and bring it to where the ''tiger's mouth'' sits just beneath the left elbow. You are now facing west.

POSTURE 29

倒攆猴(右式)

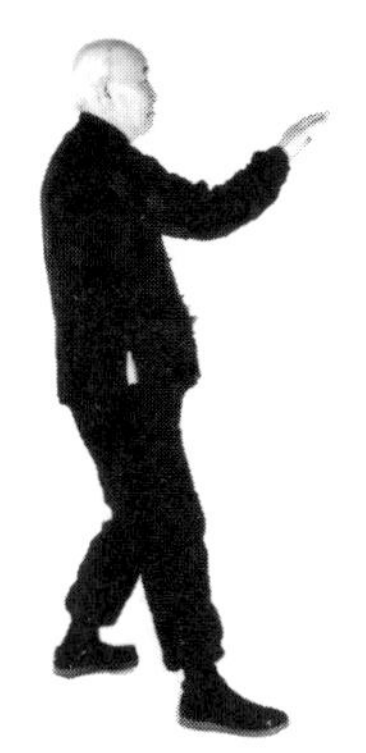

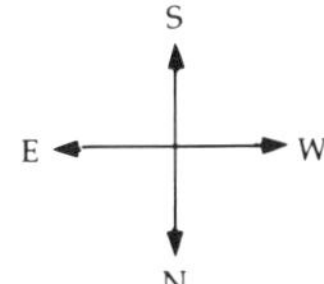

STEP BACK TO DRIVE THE MONKEY AWAY (RIGHT)

(TAO NIEN HOU, YU SHIH)

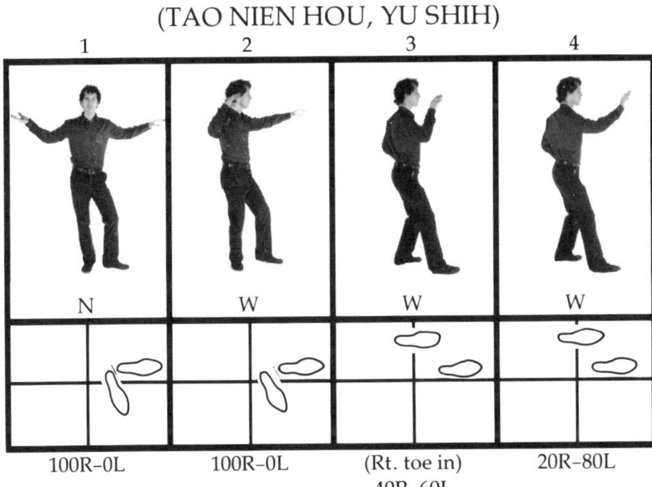

During the Counts of:

1. Turn your body to the right (facing north) and opening your right fist, palm up, circle your right hand counterclockwise, downward, backward and upward and extend it toward the east at shoulder height. At the same time turn your left hand, palm down, and extend it to the front (west) at shoulder height.
2. Turn your body to the left (to face west) and continue to circle your right hand by bringing it forward and place it beside your right ear with the palm forward and slightly downward.
3. Turn your left hand palm upward and draw it back and downward and put it beside your left thigh. Draw the right hand downward, with the elbow bent, in front of the chest with the fingers pointing slightly upwards. At the same time step back with your left foot with toes pointing directly west and shift the weight to it and curve your toes slightly inward.
4. When most of your weight has been shifted to your left foot gradually push your right hand forward with the elbow slightly bent and the palm outward. You are still facing west.

POSTURE 30

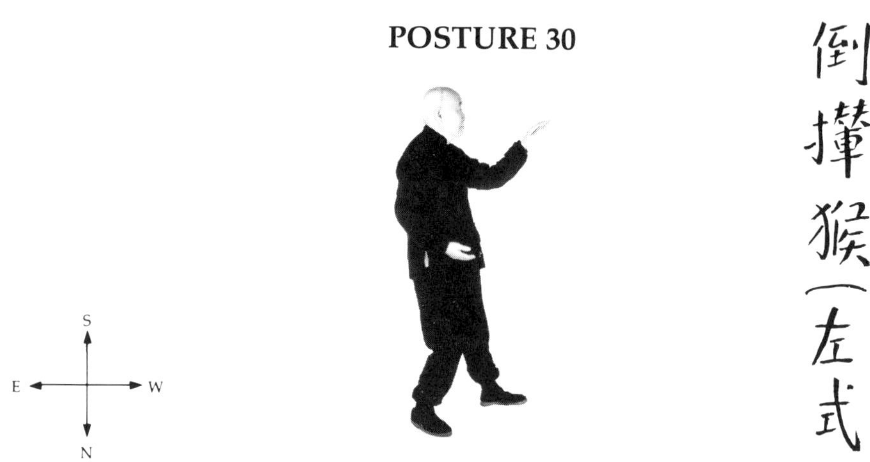

倒攆猴（左式）

STEP BACK TO DRIVE THE MONKEY AWAY (LEFT)

(TAO NIEN HOU, TSO SHIH)

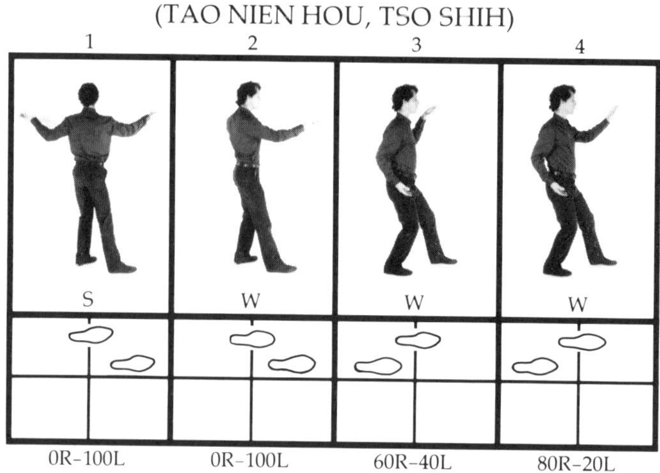

During the Counts of:

1. Turn your body to the left (to face south) and circle your left hand downward, backward and upward to extend it eastward at shoulder height with palm upward. Extend your right hand toward the west with palm downward.
2. Turn your body to the right (to face west) and bending your left arm, shift your left hand beside your left ear, with palm forward and slightly downward.
3. Turn your right hand, palm up, and draw it back and downward and put it beside your right thigh. Draw the left hand downward, with the elbow bent, in front of the chest with the fingers pointing slightly upwards. At the same time draw back your right foot and shift the weight to it with toes pointing directly forward (west).
4. Push forward with your left hand, with the elbow slightly bent and palm outward. You are still facing west.

POSTURE 31

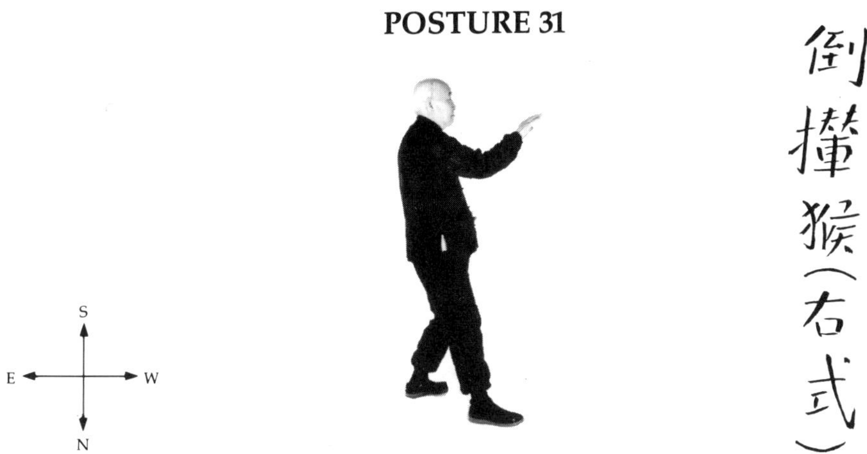

STEP BACK TO DRIVE THE MONKEY AWAY (RIGHT)

(TAO NIEN HOU, YU SHIH)

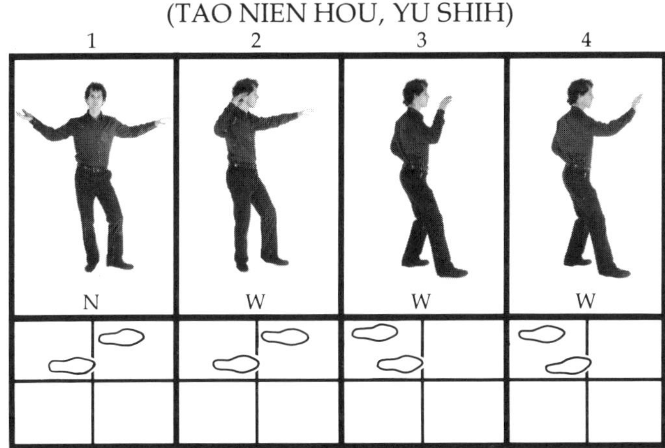

This posture is the same as posture #29 except the feet always point west. Therefore, there is no toe in on beat #3.

POSTURE 32

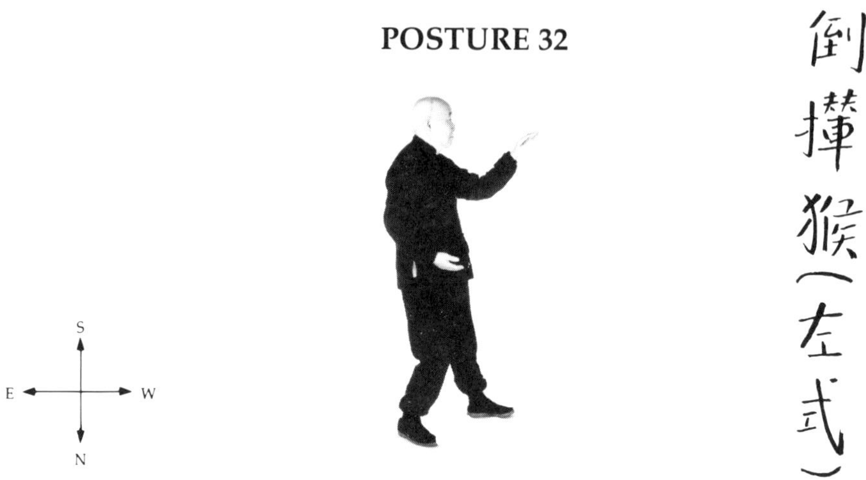

STEP BACK TO DRIVE THE MONKEY AWAY (LEFT)

(TAO NIEN HOU, TSO SHIH)

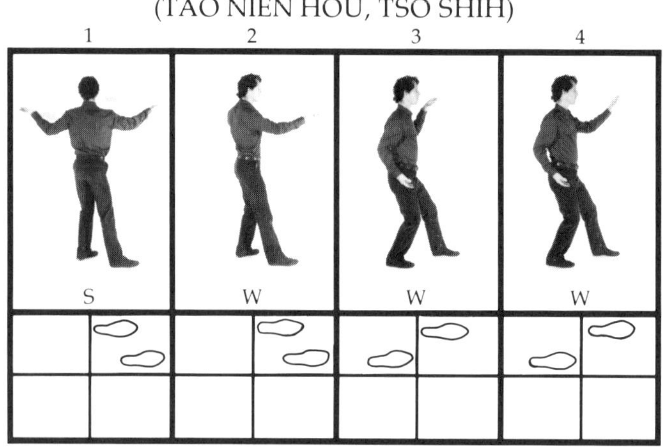

This posture is the same as posture #30.

POSTURE 33

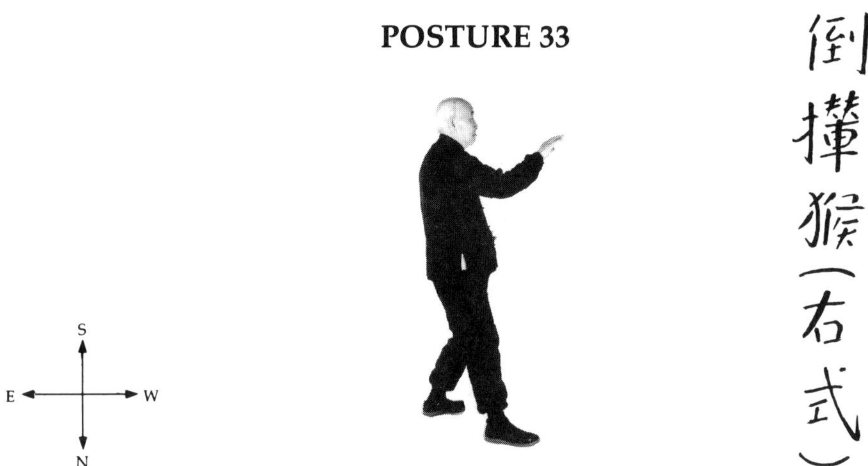

STEP BACK TO DRIVE THE MONKEY AWAY (RIGHT)

(TAO NIEN HOU, YU SHIH)

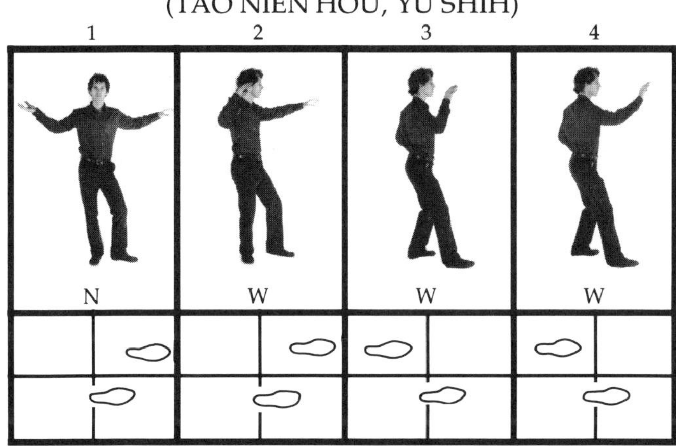

This posture is the same as posture #29 except the feet always point west. Therefore, there is no toe in.

POSTURE 34

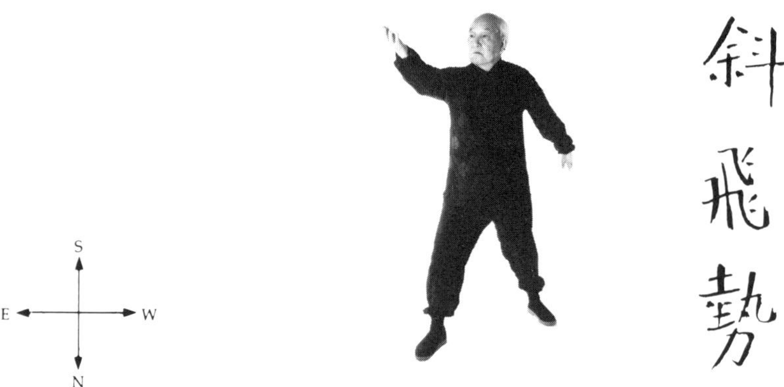

DIAGONAL FLYING POSTURE

(HSIEH FEI SHIH)

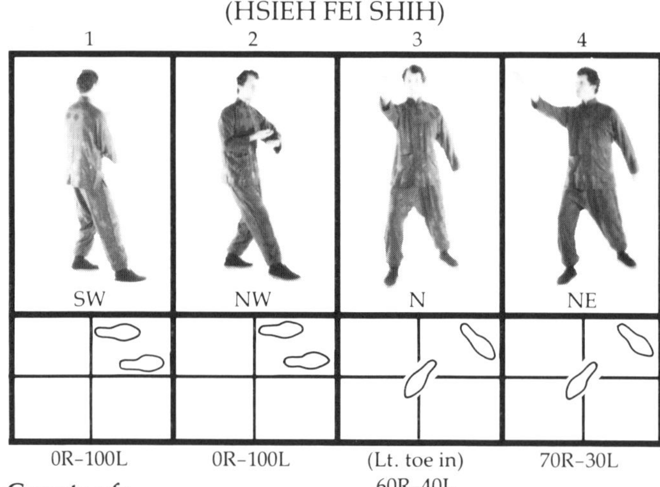

During the Counts of:

1. Turn your body slightly to the left (to face southwest) and lower your right hand and raise your left hand. Most of the weight is on the left leg.
2. Continue to lower your right hand, turning it palm up, and stop it in front of (and near) your left thigh. Raise your left hand, palm down and stop it in front of the left side of your chest so that your hands simulate holding a ball. Turn your body to the right. Bring the arm (right) from beneath the left armpit to the back of the left arm.
3. Continue to turn your body to the right and take one big step with your right foot to the far right (northeast) with the heel touching first. Sweep the right arm across to the right with the turn of the body. The palm is in an upward position. Shift the weight to the right leg and turn the left foot slightly inward, pivoting on the heel.
4. Shift 70% of your weight to your right foot. The right arm continues to move in a diagonal upward position past and above head level as the body turns to the northeast. At the same time draw back and extend your left hand behind your left thigh in a diagonally downward position, (fingers pointing south-west). You are now facing northeast.

POSTURE 35

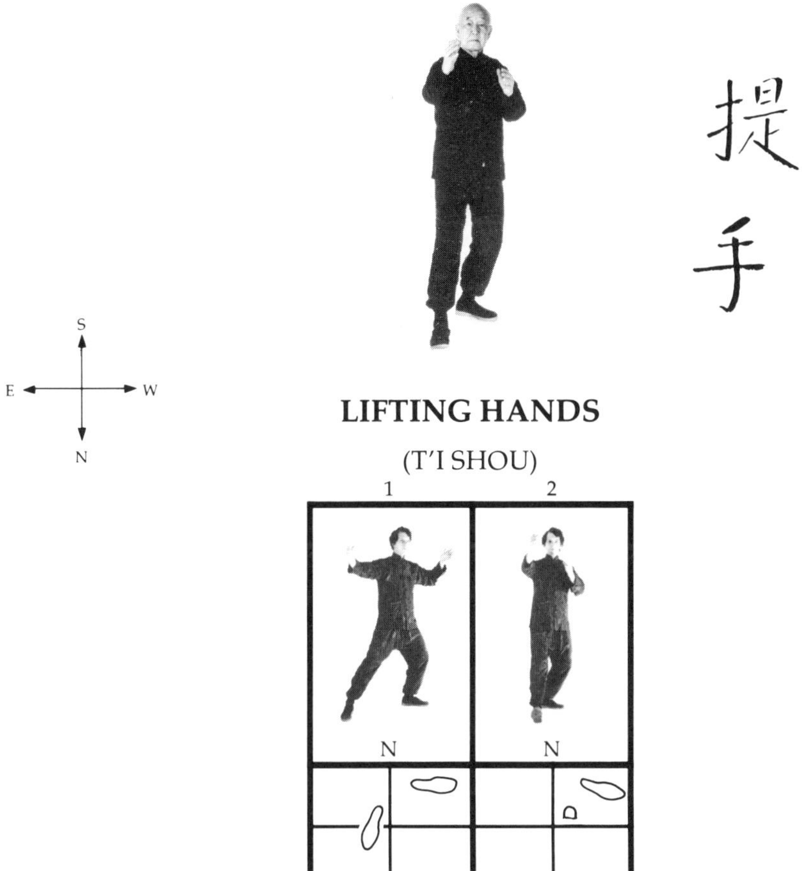

LIFTING HANDS

(T'I SHOU)

During the Counts of:

1. As you turn your torso leftward (to face north), pick up your left foot and set it down slightly outward (pointing NW) and shift the weight to it. At the same time turn your palms inward so that they face each other.
2. This beat is the same as the respective beat of posture #9.

POSTURE 36

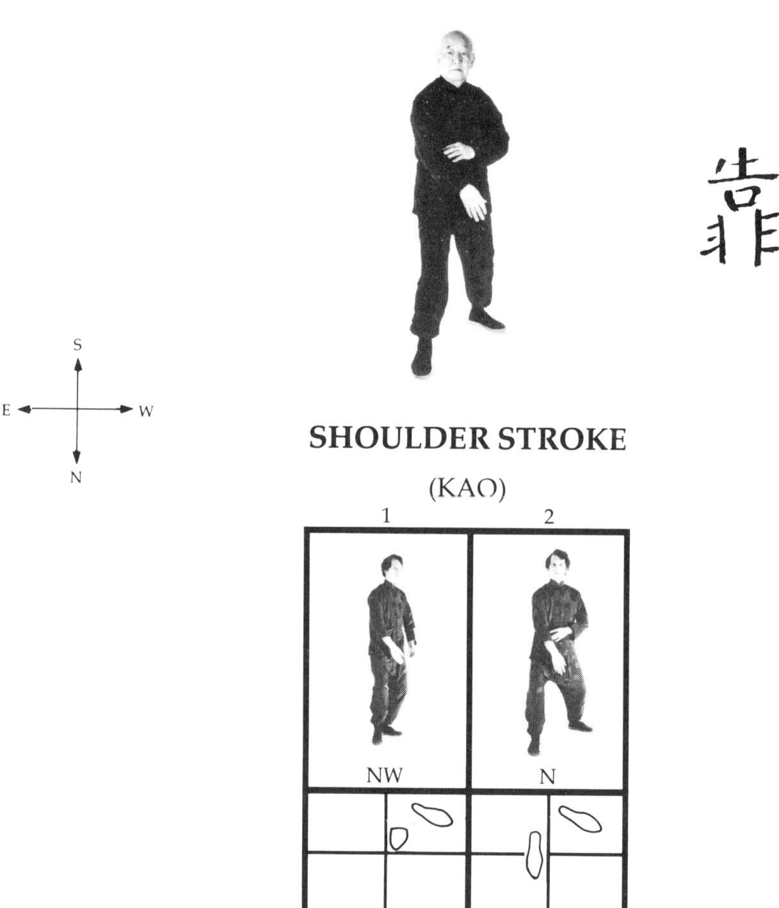

SHOULDER STROKE

(KAO)

This posture is the same as posture #10.

POSTURE 37

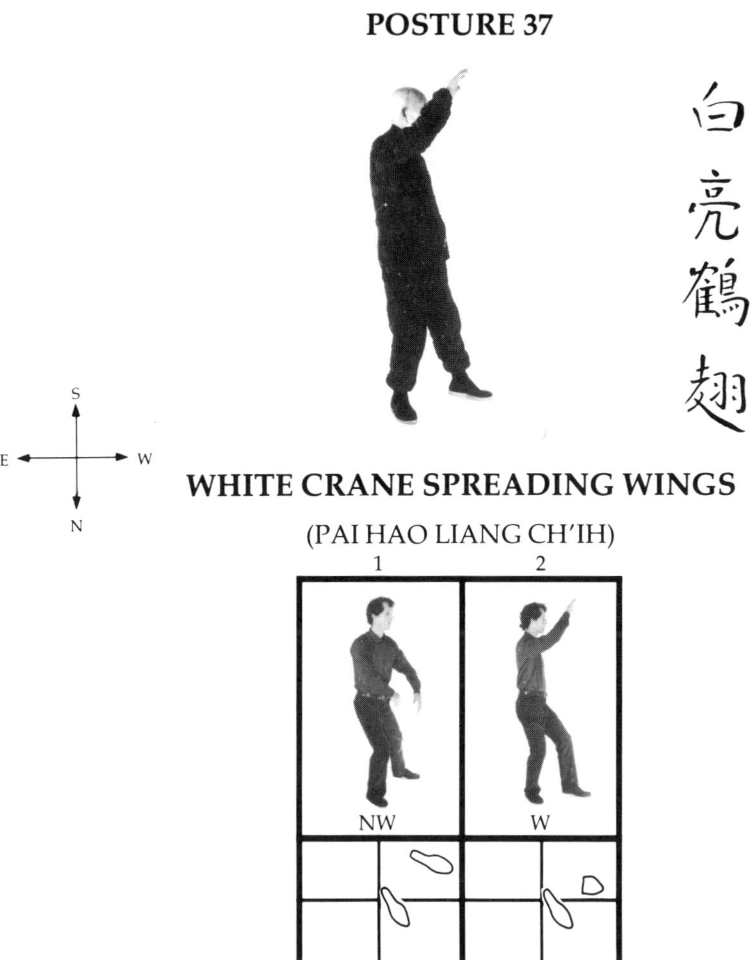

WHITE CRANE SPREADING WINGS

(PAI HAO LIANG CH'IH)

This posture is the same as posture #11.

POSTURE 38

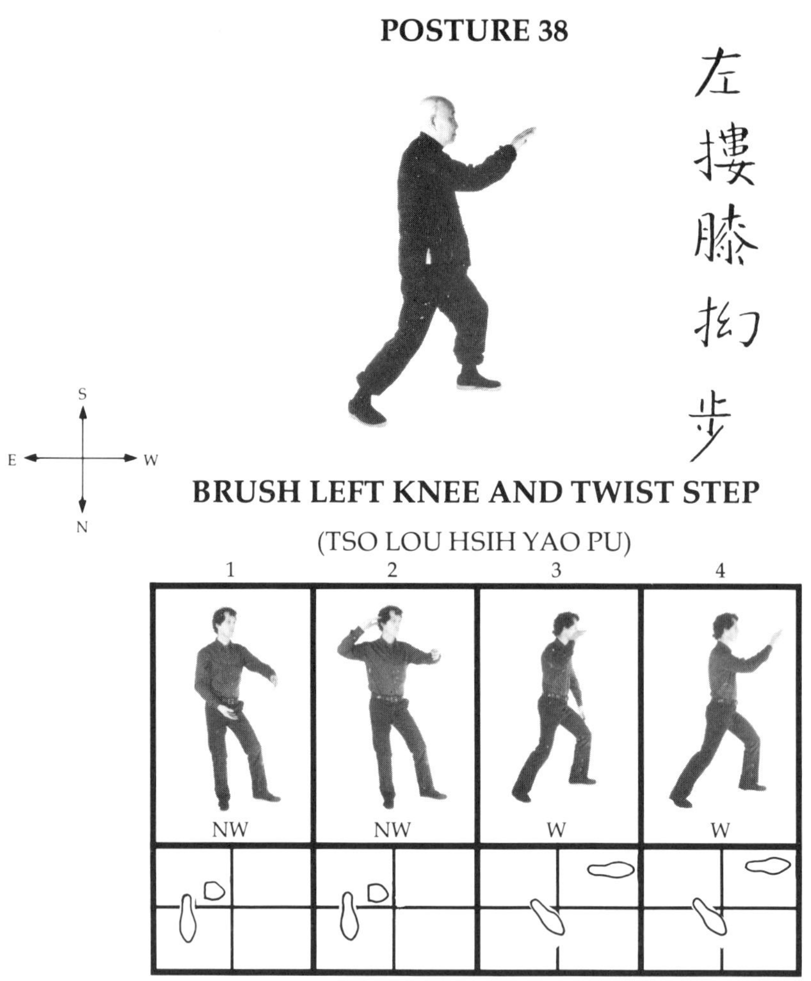

BRUSH LEFT KNEE AND TWIST STEP

(TSO LOU HSIH YAO PU)

This posture is the same as posture #12.

POSTURE 39

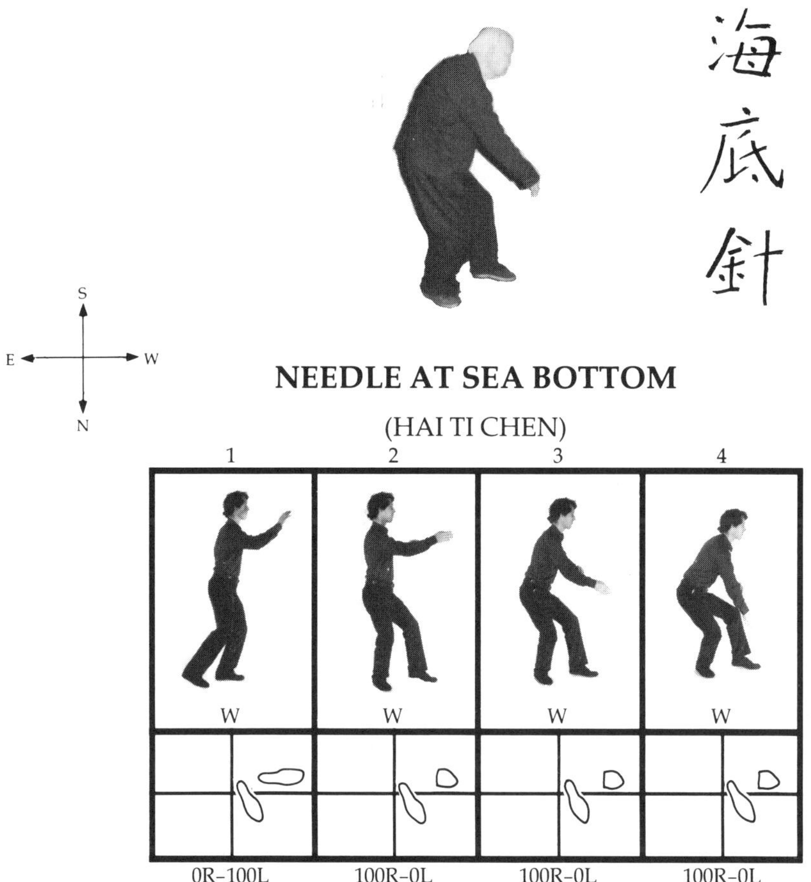

NEEDLE AT SEA BOTTOM

(HAI TI CHEN)

1	2	3	4
W	W	W	W
0R–100L	100R–0L	100R–0L	100R–0L

During the Counts of:

1. Pick up your right foot and set it down with toes turned slightly outward (NW) and begin to shift the weight to it.
2. Stretch your right hand forward at chest level with palm facing south, fingers pointing forward (west) and put your left hand by the crook of your right forearm. At the same time shift your left foot slightly backward and to the right with the toes touching the ground. (This is done after all the weight has been shifted to the right leg).
3. Gradually lower your right hand (with the left hand still lightly attached) and lower your body by bending your right knee.
4. Continue to lower your right hand and your body so that your right fingers point directly to the ground below your right knee (without bending at the waist). You are still facing west.

POSTURE 40

扇通背

S
E W
N

FAN PENETRATES THE BACK

(SHAN T'UNG PEI)

1	2	3	4
W	W	W	W
100R–0L	100R–0L	40R–60L	30R–70L

During the Counts of:

1. Raise your body and raise your right hand to chest level with the palm facing south and with your left hand still attached to the crook of your right forearm.
2. Continue to raise your right hand and bring it near you right temple with the palm outward and elbow bent. At the same time move your left hand forward with the palm outward and elbow bent.
3. Take a half step forward and leftward with your left foot (with heel touching first) and shift the weight to it.
4. Gradually push forward with your left palm with the elbow slightly bent shifting 70% of your weight to the left foot. You are still facing west.

POSTURE 41

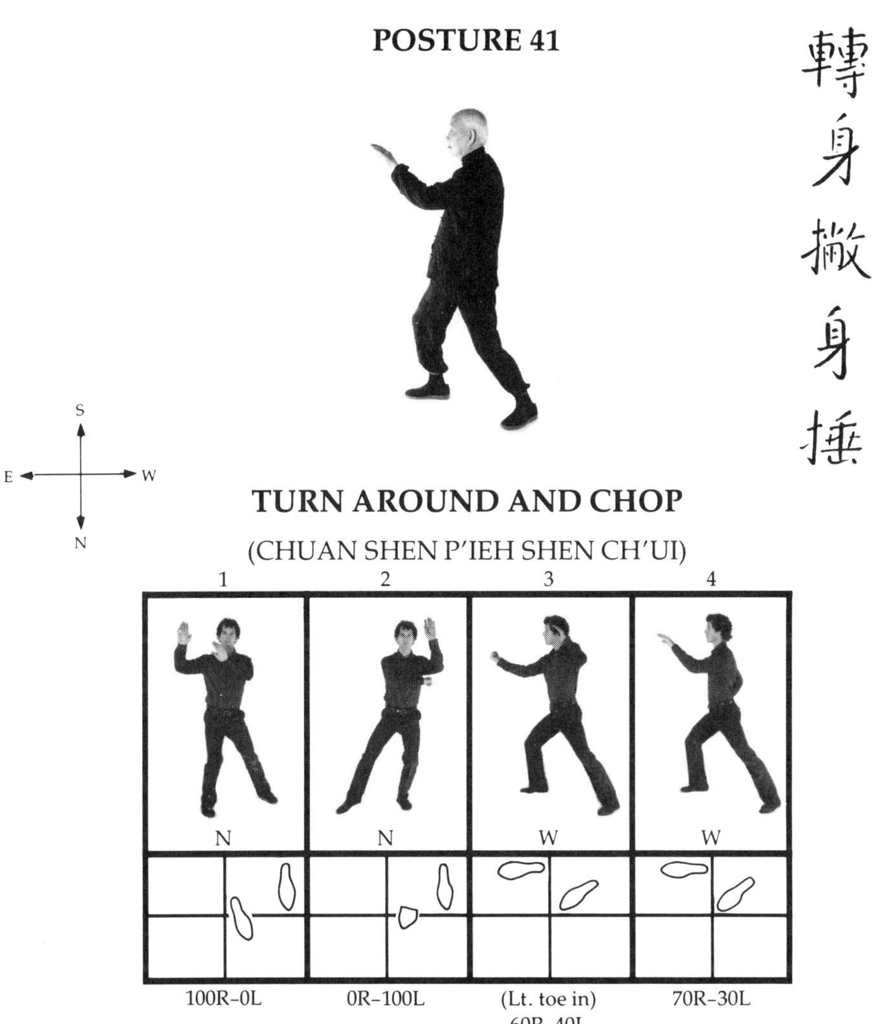

TURN AROUND AND CHOP

(CHUAN SHEN P'IEH SHEN CH'UI)

During the Counts of:

1. Circle your hands clockwise to the right, turning your body in the same direction (north) while shifting your weight to the right foot. At the same time curve your left foot inward facing north.
2. Continue to turn your hands clockwise, downward, leftward and upward until your left hand is near your left temple, with palm outward and elbow bent, and your right is clenched into a fist with knuckles up, in the front of the left side of the body. At the same time shift your weight to the left foot and let the right heel be brought off the ground.
3. Turn your body to the right (east) and raise your right foot to take a half step to the forward right direction with the heel touching first and toes pointing east. Make your right fist circle upward vertically to the right and chop down toward the southeast, and then withdraw it to the right side of your waist with knuckles down. At the same time gradually shift your weight to your right foot and curve your left toes slightly inward. (Note: The picture shown

for this count is halfway through the movements described for count #3, to show the actual chop.)

4. Shift 70% of your weight to your right foot and lastly push forward with your left palm. You are now facing east.

POSTURE 42

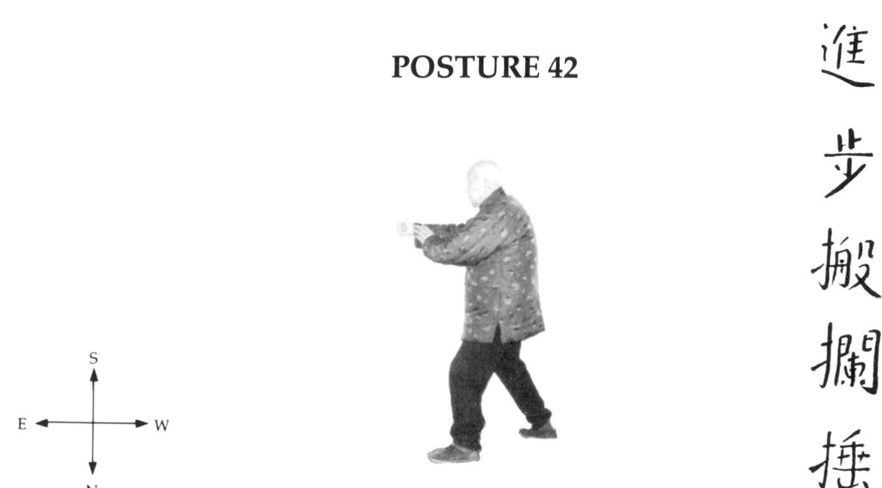

STEP FORWARD, DEFLECT DOWNWARD, INTERCEPT AND PUNCH

(CHIN PU PAN LAN CH'UI)

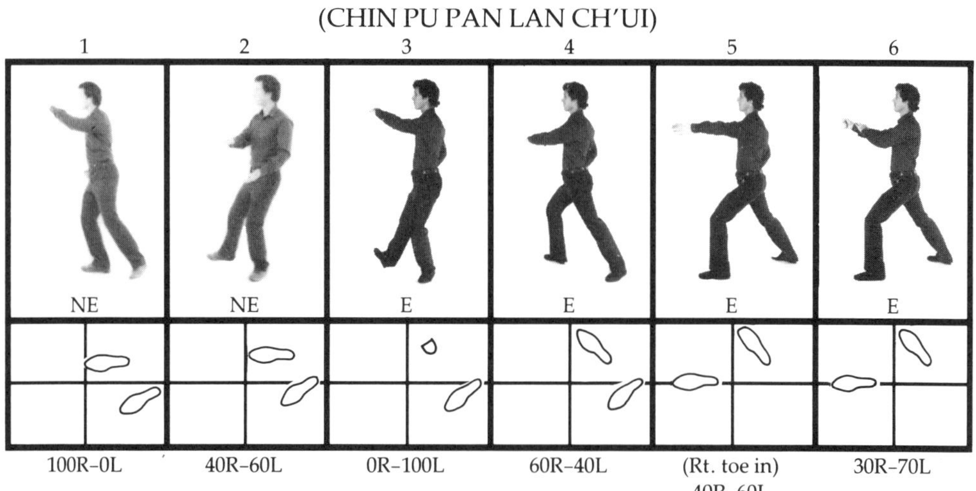

This posture is the same as posture #20 except:

1. Pick up your left foot and set it down (pointing NE).
2. Turn body to NE.
3. Toes point SE (right foot).

Beats 4, 5 and 6 are the same as the respective beats of posture #20.

POSTURE 43

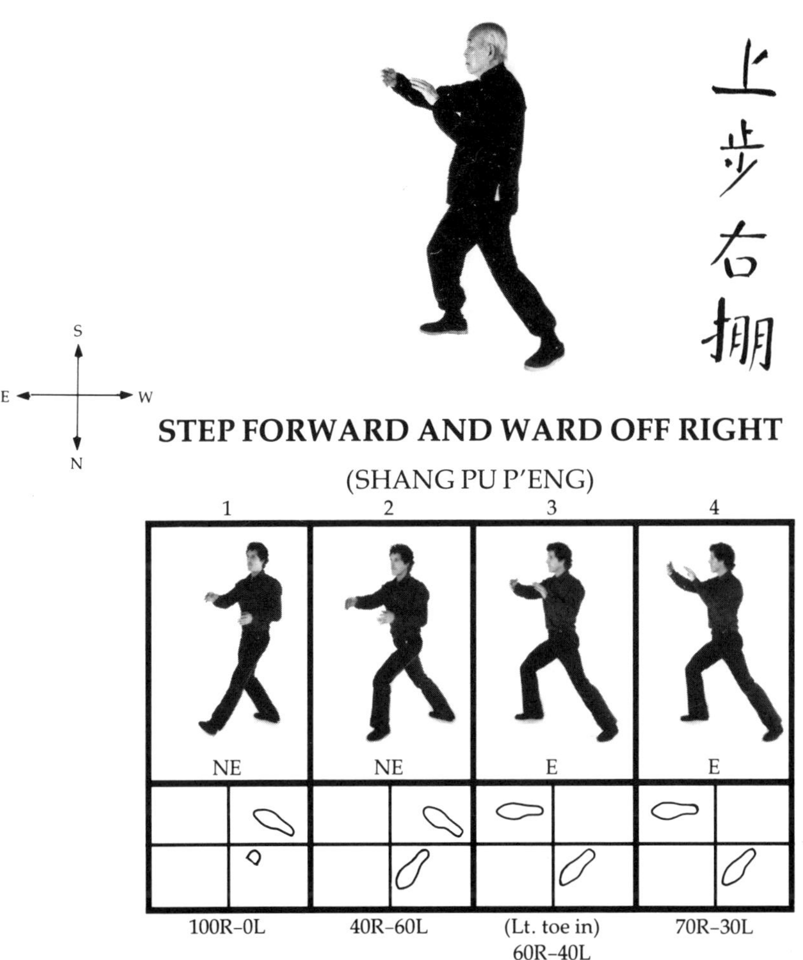

STEP FORWARD AND WARD OFF RIGHT

(SHANG PU P'ENG)

During the Counts of:

1. Shift your weight to your right foot. Turn your body to the left (to face NE). Open the right fist and let the arm turn with the body to the left. Let your left hand turn with the body also. Raise the left toes and turn the foot slightly outward to the left. At the same time turn your body slightly to the left (to face NE).
2. Gradually shift your weight to the left foot.

Beats 3 and 4 are the same as the respective beats of posture #4.

POSTURE 44

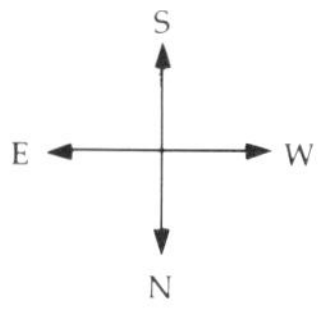

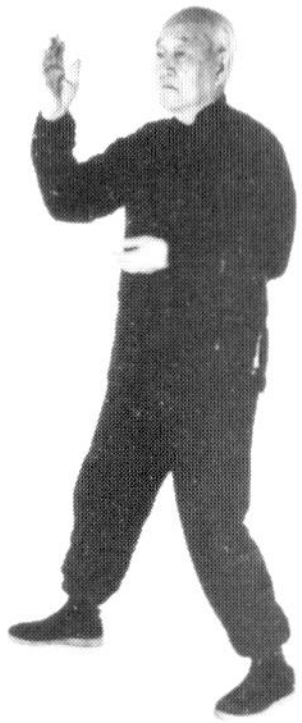

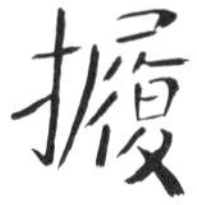

S
E W
N

ROLL BACK

(LÜ)

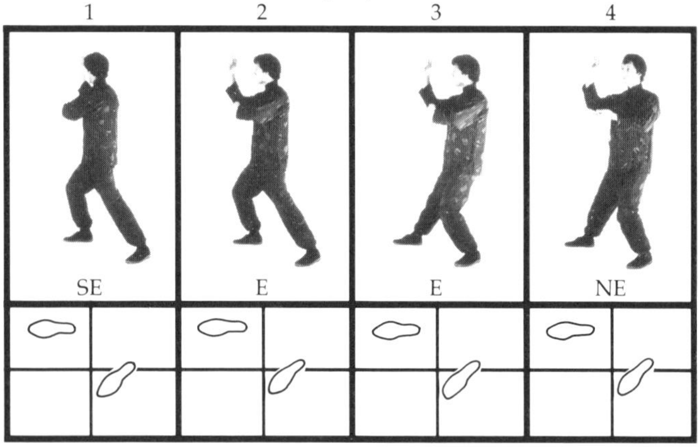

1	2	3	4
SE	E	E	NE

This posture is the same as posture #5.

POSTURE 45

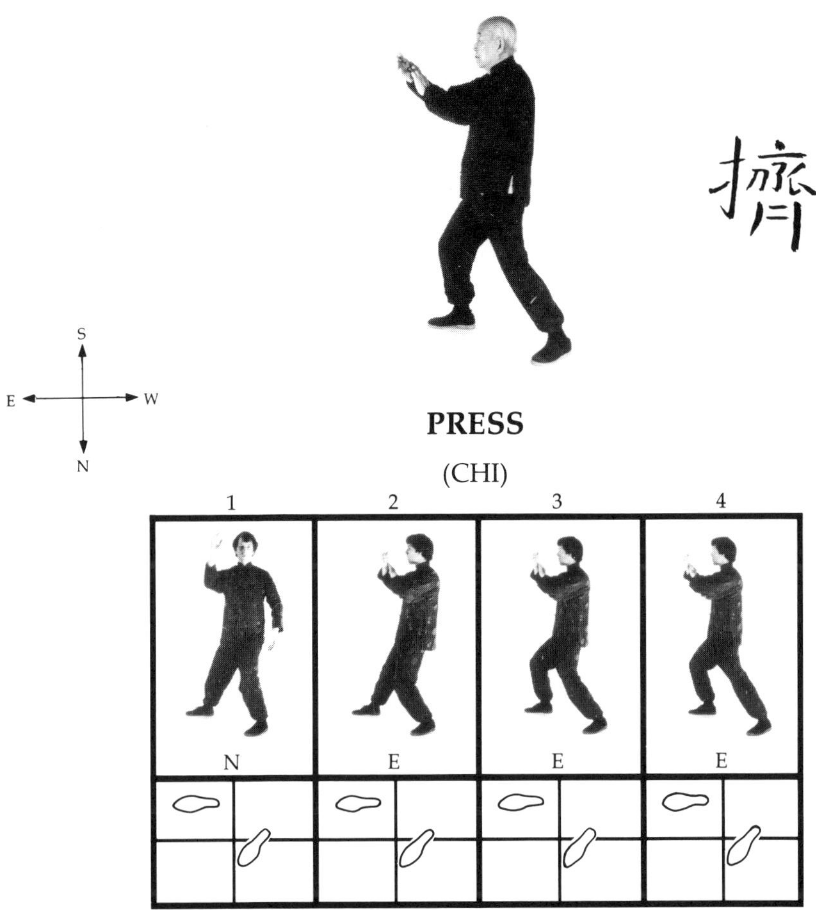

PRESS

(CHI)

This posture is the same as posture #6.

POSTURE 46

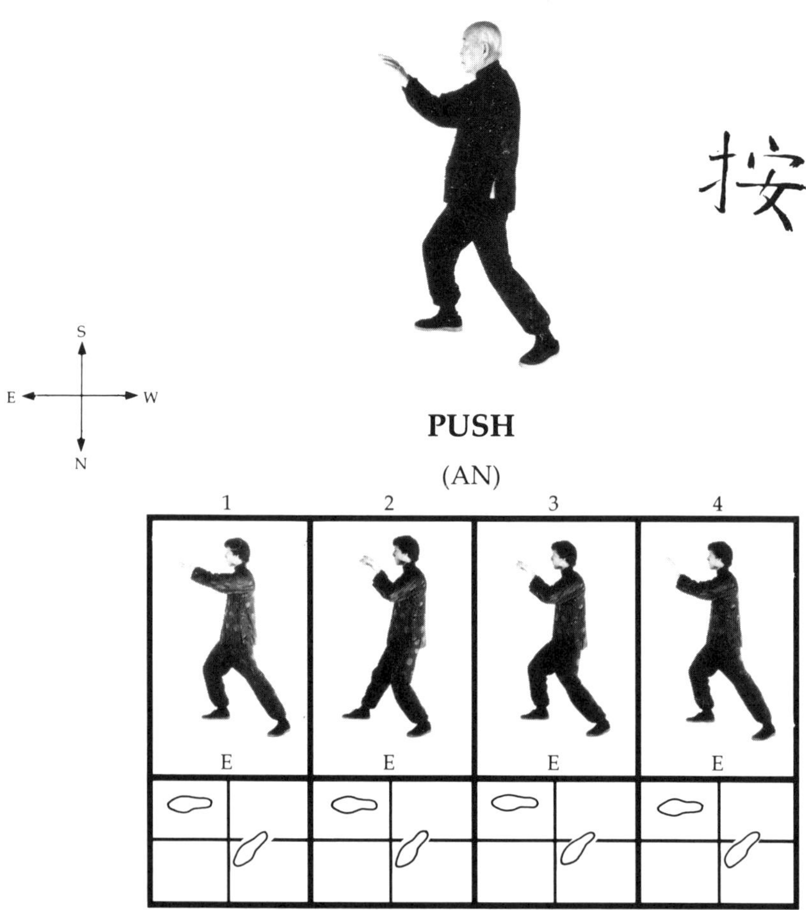

PUSH

(AN)

This posture is the same as posture #7.

POSTURE 47

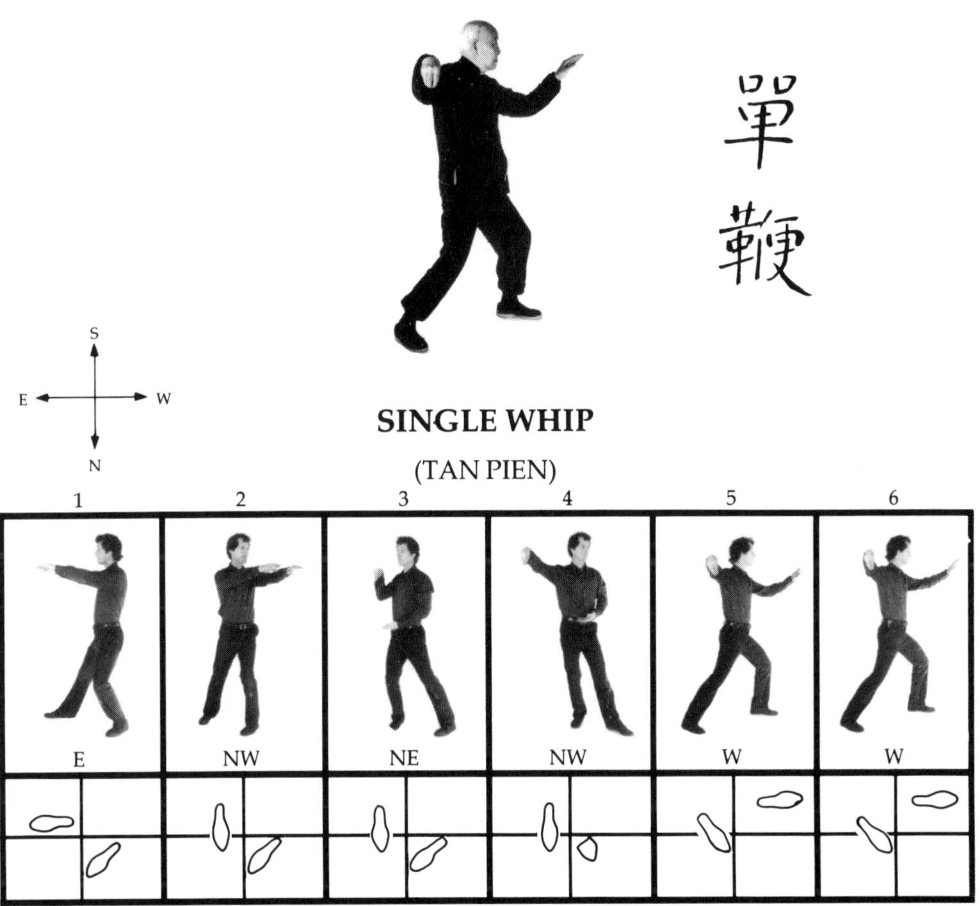

SINGLE WHIP

(TAN PIEN)

This posture is the same as posture #8.

POSTURE 48

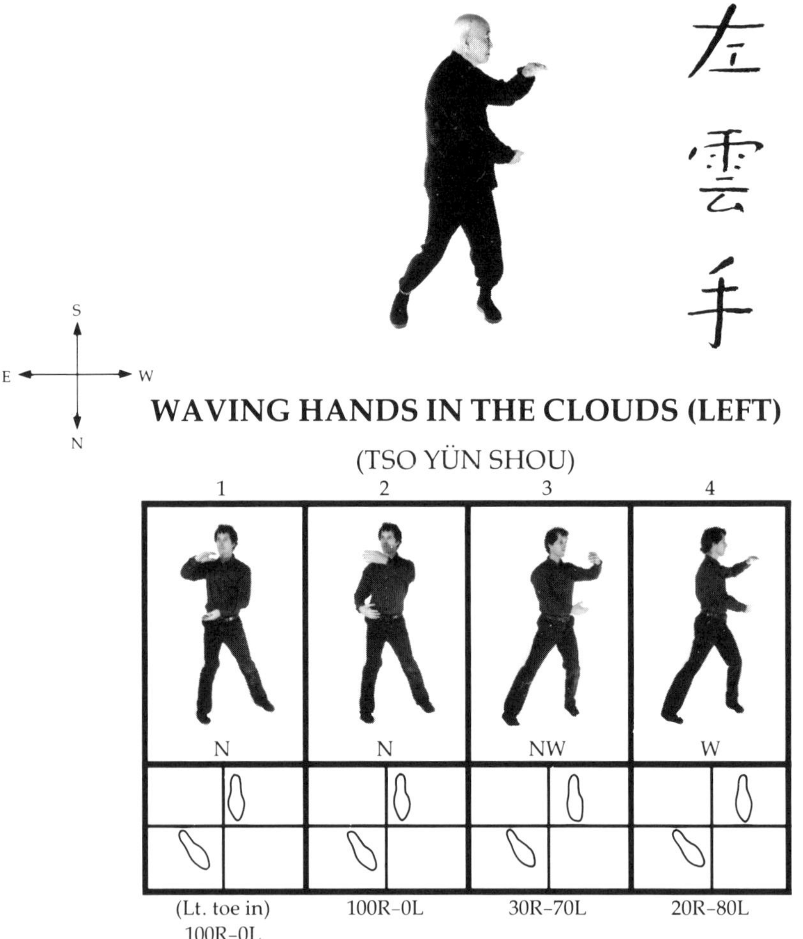

WAVING HANDS IN THE CLOUDS (LEFT)

(TSO YÜN SHOU)

During the Counts of:

1. Open your right "hook" hand and turn your right hand, palm down, drawing it back in front near your neck while turning your torso to the right (to face north). Shift your weight to the right foot, turn your left foot inward (pointing north), and turn your left hand, palm up, beside your abdomen. Now your hands simulate holding a ball.
2. Lower your right hand near to your abdomen with palm inward and raise your left hand to neck height with palm facing you. The weight is still on the right foot.
3. Turn your torso gradually to the left (to face NW) and shift the weight to the left foot.
4. Continue to turn your torso together with both of your hands to the left. Shift all the weight to the left foot until your right hand, palm up, is near your abdomen and the left hand, palm down, is near your neck. You, again, are simulating the holding of a ball and are facing west.

POSTURE 49

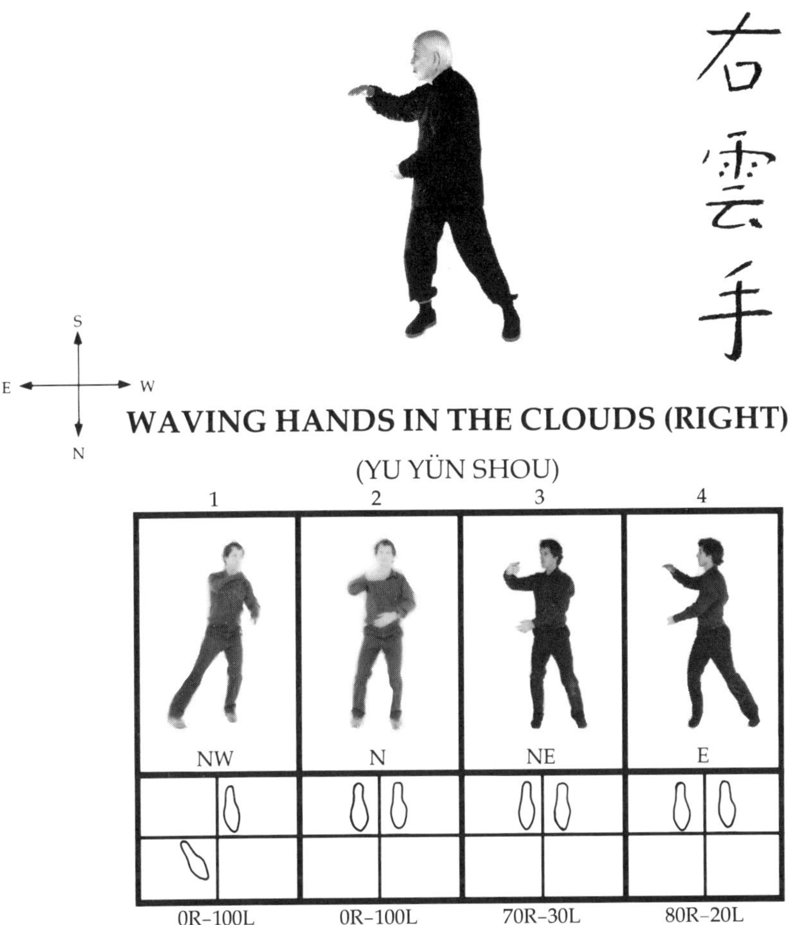

WAVING HANDS IN THE CLOUDS (RIGHT)

(YU YÜN SHOU)

During the Counts of:

1. Turn the torso to the right (NW), lowering the left hand so that the palm faces the body. The right hand rises to neck level with this palm also facing the body. Both hands are over the left thigh.
2. Draw your right foot back in line with your left foot with the toes pointing north (the distance between the feet should be equal to shoulder width).
3. Continue to turn your torso and circle your hands to the right (NE) and gradually shift your weight to your right foot.
4. Continue to turn your torso and hands to the right until you face east. Your right hand, palm down, is near your neck, and your left hand, palm up is near your abdomen and under your right hand. Again you simulate holding a ball. You are now facing east.

POSTURE 50

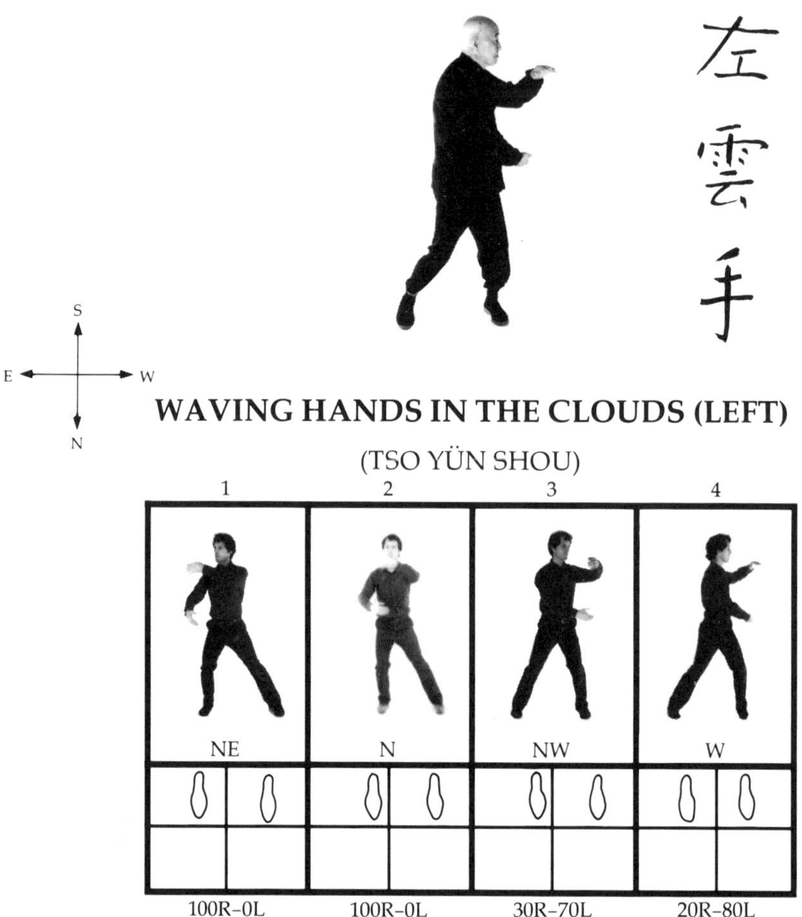

WAVING HANDS IN THE CLOUDS (LEFT)

(TSO YÜN SHOU)

During the Counts of:

1. Take a one-half step sideways to the left with your left foot. Turn your torso gradually to the left (NE) and at the same time circle your hands to the left. The left hand circles upward and the right hand downward.
2. Continue to turn your torso and hands to the left until you face north. Your left hand, palm in, is at the level of your neck, and your right hand, palm in, is at the level of your abdomen while the weight is still on the right foot.

Beats 3 and 4 are the same as the respective beats of posture #48.

POSTURE 51

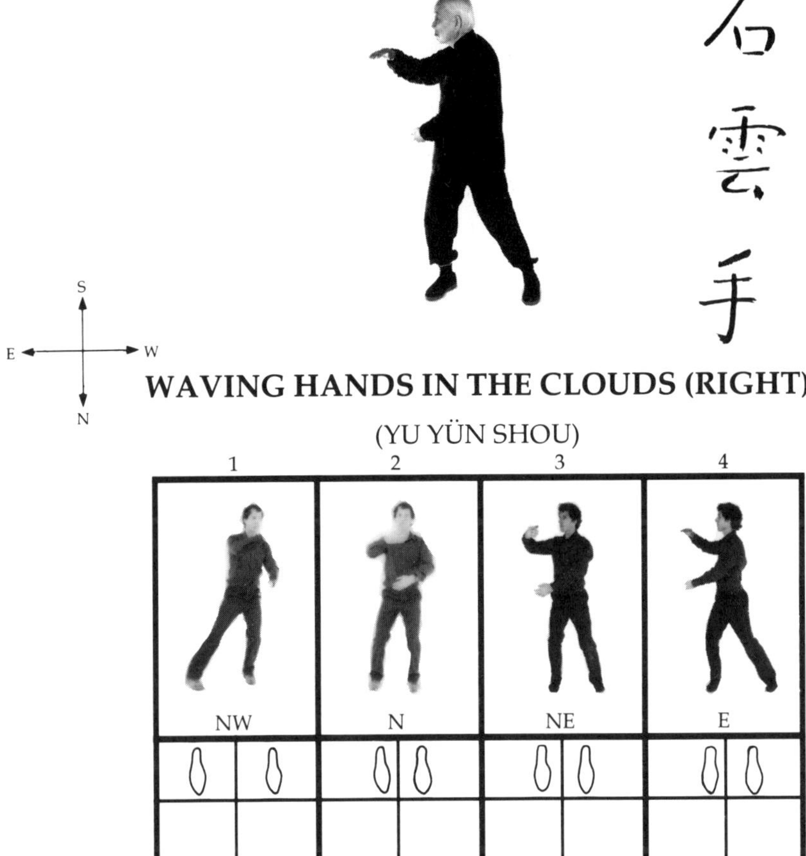

WAVING HANDS IN THE CLOUDS (RIGHT)

(YU YÜN SHOU)

This posture is the same as posture #49.

POSTURE 52

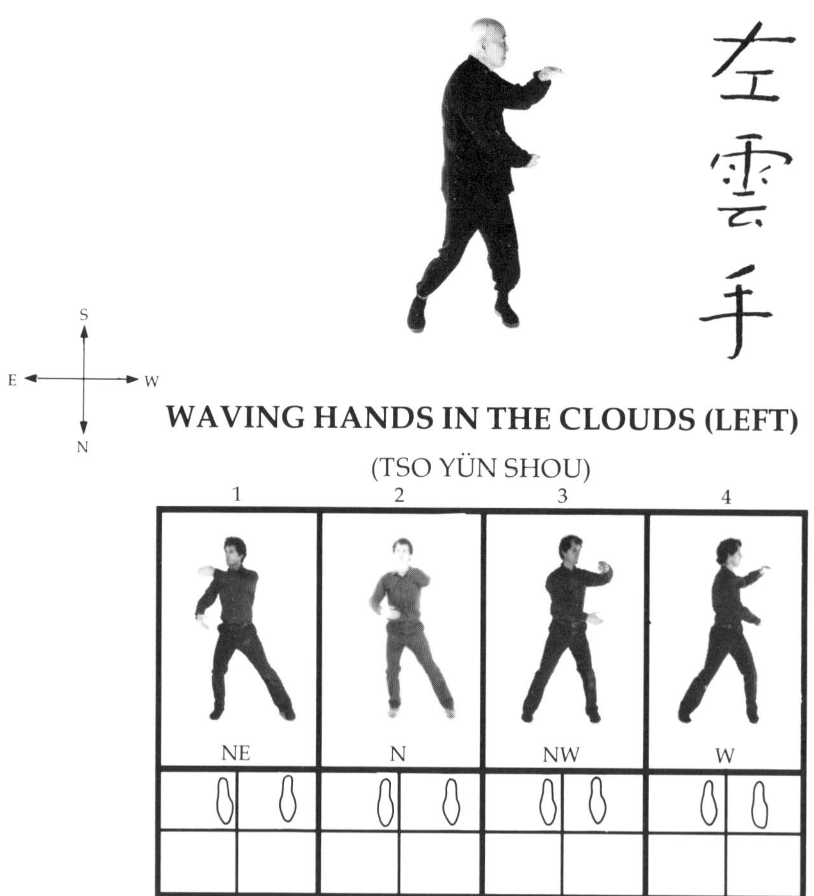

WAVING HANDS IN THE CLOUDS (LEFT)

(TSO YÜN SHOU)

This posture is the same as posture #50.

POSTURE 53

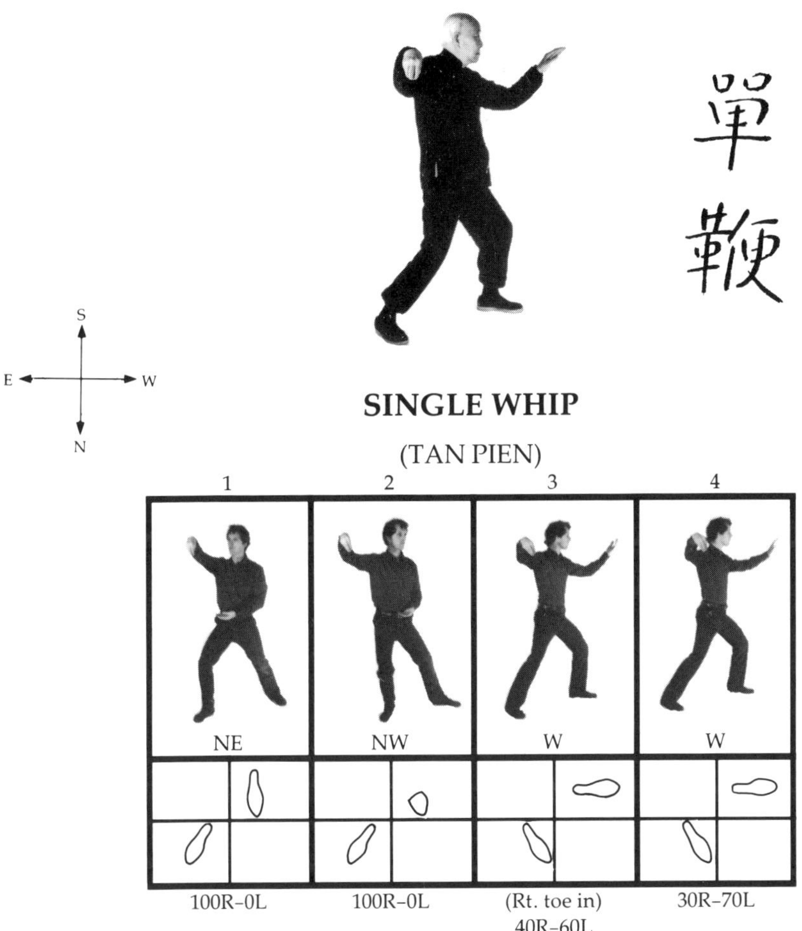

SINGLE WHIP

(TAN PIEN)

During the Counts of:

1. Take a step to the forward right direction (NE) with your right foot, (heel touching first) and shift the weight to it. Gradually turn your torso to the right. Make a "hook hand" with the fingers pointing down and extend the hand to the NE. At the same time lower your left hand, palm up, near your chest.
2. Gradually turn your torso to the left (NW) with left heel up and toes pointing west.
3. Continue to turn your torso to the left (west) and step forward and to the left with your left heel touching first. Shift the weight to this leg. Raise your left hand in front of you at the level of your eyes with palm inward and turn your right foot slightly inward.
4. Shift 70% of your weight to your left foot. Turn your left palm outward as your eyes, which have accompanied the gradual turn, look across the fingers of your left extended hand. You are now facing west.

POSTURE 54

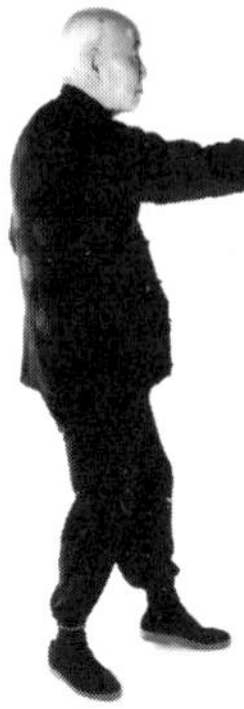

高探馬

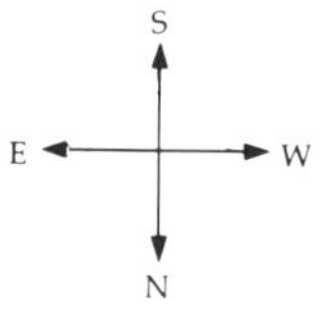

E W S N

HIGH PAT ON HORSE

(KAO T'AN MA)

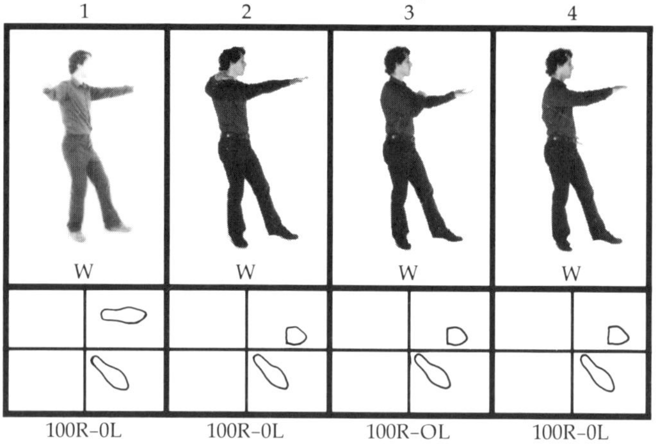

1	2	3	4
W	W	W	W
100R-0L	100R-0L	100R-OL	100R-0L

During the Counts of:

1. Pick up your right foot and lower it with the foot turned slightly outward. Shift the weight to it, bending the right knee slightly.
2. Shift your left foot slightly rightward and backward with the heel raised and toes touching the ground.
   Open your right "hook hand".
3. Turn the left palm upward. The right hand bends so that the fingers touch the left bicep.
4. Draw your left hand backward and extend your right hand forward until your left hand is near your abdomen (with palm up) and your right is in front and over your left hand (with palm downward) with the elbow slightly bent. You still face west.

POSTURE 55

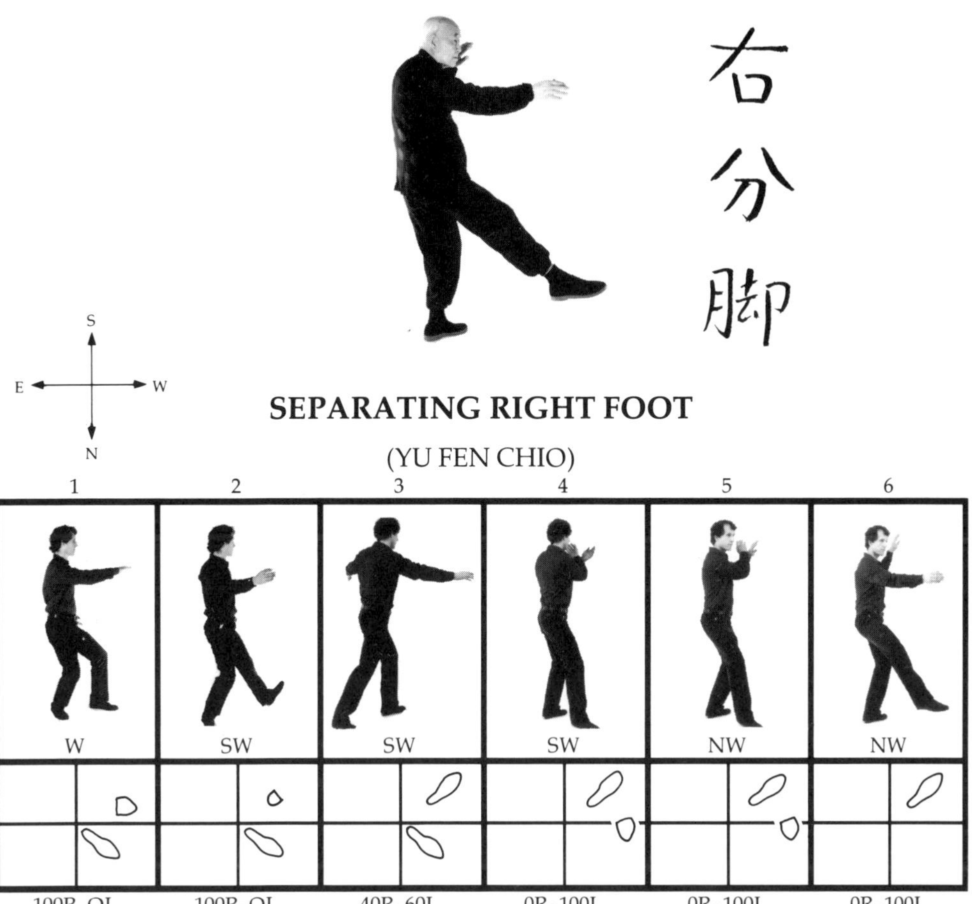

SEPARATING RIGHT FOOT

(YU FEN CHIO)

During the Counts of:

1. Sink weight onto right leg.
2. Step with your left foot to the forward left direction. Only the heel touches with the toes pointing southwest.
3. Shift your weight to the left foot and gradually separate and circle your hands in opposite directions, upwards and sideways.
4. Continue to circle your hands downward and upward until the wrists join with the right hand outside of the left hand and both palms face inward. At the same time shift your right foot near your left foot with the heel up and toes pointing towards the ground.
5. Turn your palms outward and gradually turn your body to the right (to face NW).
6. Separate your hands in the opposite directions while at the same time kicking your right foot forward (NW). Keep your right foot straight with your right hand aligned to your right foot. The gaze of your eyes and your right hand are focused on the intended object. Your left arm has the elbow bent and fingers pointing upward so as to maintain balance. You are now facing NW.

POSTURE 56

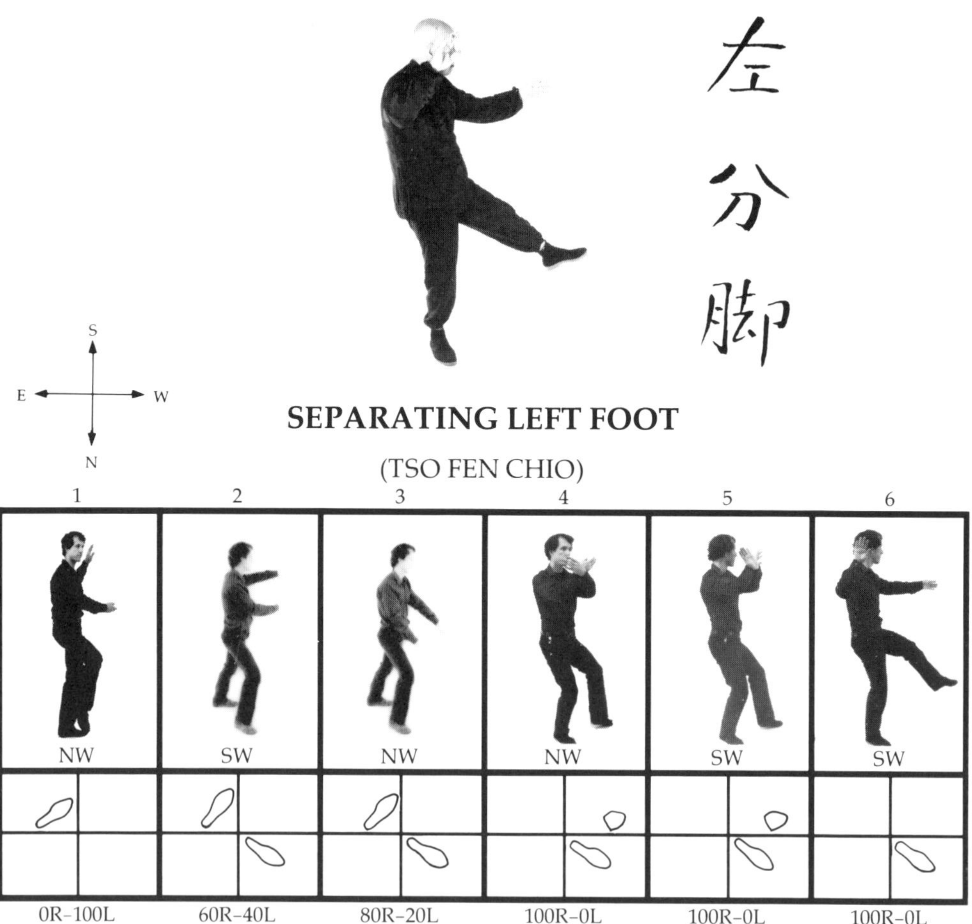

SEPARATING LEFT FOOT

(TSO FEN CHIO)

During the Counts of:

1. Bend the right knee with foot suspended in the air and toes pointing down, and at the same time withdraw the right hand with palm upward.
2. Lower your right foot and step one full step to the NW with heel touching first; shift the weight to it. At the same time stretch the left hand to the SW with palm down and turn your body slightly to the left (SW).
3. Circle both hands counterclockwise to the NE and turn your body slightly to the right (NW).
4. Join the two hands in a slanting cross shape in front of your chest with palms inward and left hand outside of the right hand. Slide the left foot to the right, moving on the toe which points southwest.
5. Turn the palms outward and turn the body slightly to the left (SW).
6. Separate your hands in the opposite directions while simultaneously kicking forward with the tip of your left foot. Keep your left foot straight with the instep and your left hand aligned to your left foot. The gaze of your eyes and your left hand are focused on the intended object. Your right arm has the elbow bent and fingers pointing upward so as to maintain balance. You are now facing southwest.

POSTURE 57

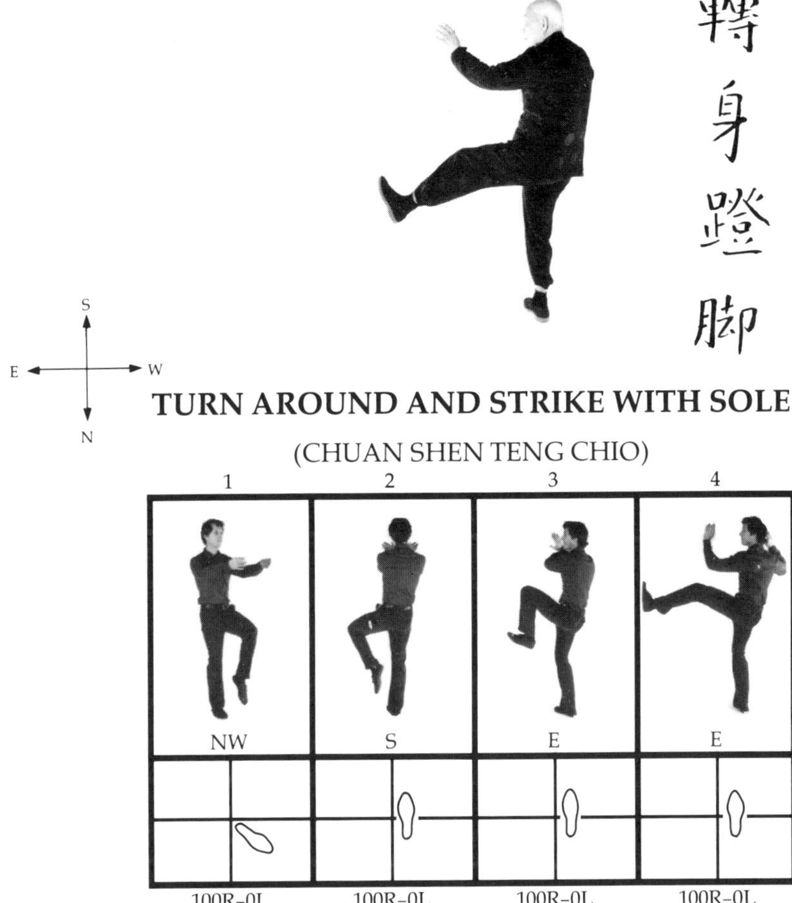

TURN AROUND AND STRIKE WITH SOLE

(CHUAN SHEN TENG CHIO)

During the Counts of:

1. Withdraw your left hand near your chest and withdraw your left leg with knee bent and foot suspended in the air. At the same time turn your torso slightly to the right (NW) and stretch your hands to the same direction with palms facing one another.
2. Swing your body by turning on your right heel to the left with the toes facing south. Your right hand circles counterclockwise when it meets and joins the left hand. The left hand is inside of the right hand, thus forming a slanting cross (body is facing south).
3. Turn your palms outward as you gradually turn your torso to the left (east) and raise your left knee with the toes slightly upward.
4. Kick forward with the sole of your left foot with toes upward while chopping forward with your left hand at the level of your nose. Your right arm is bent at the elbow with fingers pointing upward so as to maintain balance. You are now facing east.

POSTURE 58

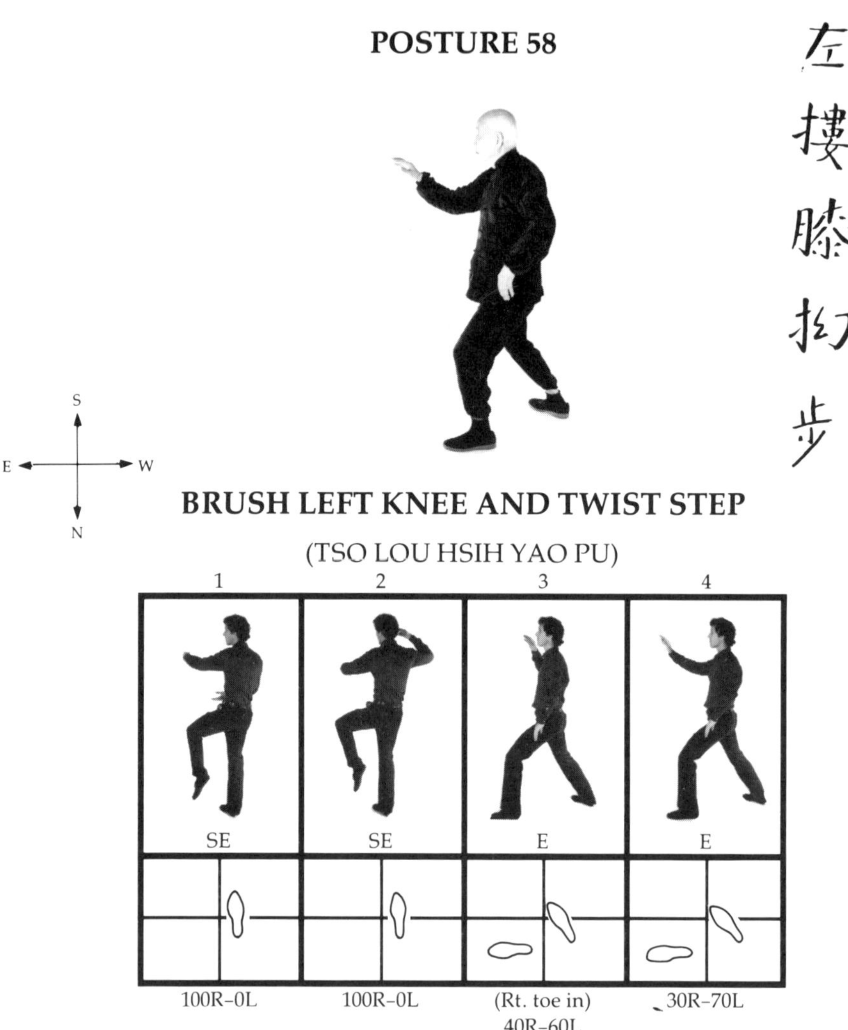

BRUSH LEFT KNEE AND TWIST STEP

(TSO LOU HSIH YAO PU)

During the Counts of: (Same as posture #12 except as indicated).

1. Lower your left hand near your chest and left leg with the knee bent. The foot is still suspended in the air while you turn your torso slightly to the right (SE).
2. Continue to turn your torso to the right (southeast) and bring the right hand up in a circling movement by the right ear. The left arm bends slightly while it turns rightward with the body: the palm faces the body.
3. Same as posture 12, beat 3, but facing east.
4. Same as posture 12, beat 4, but facing east.

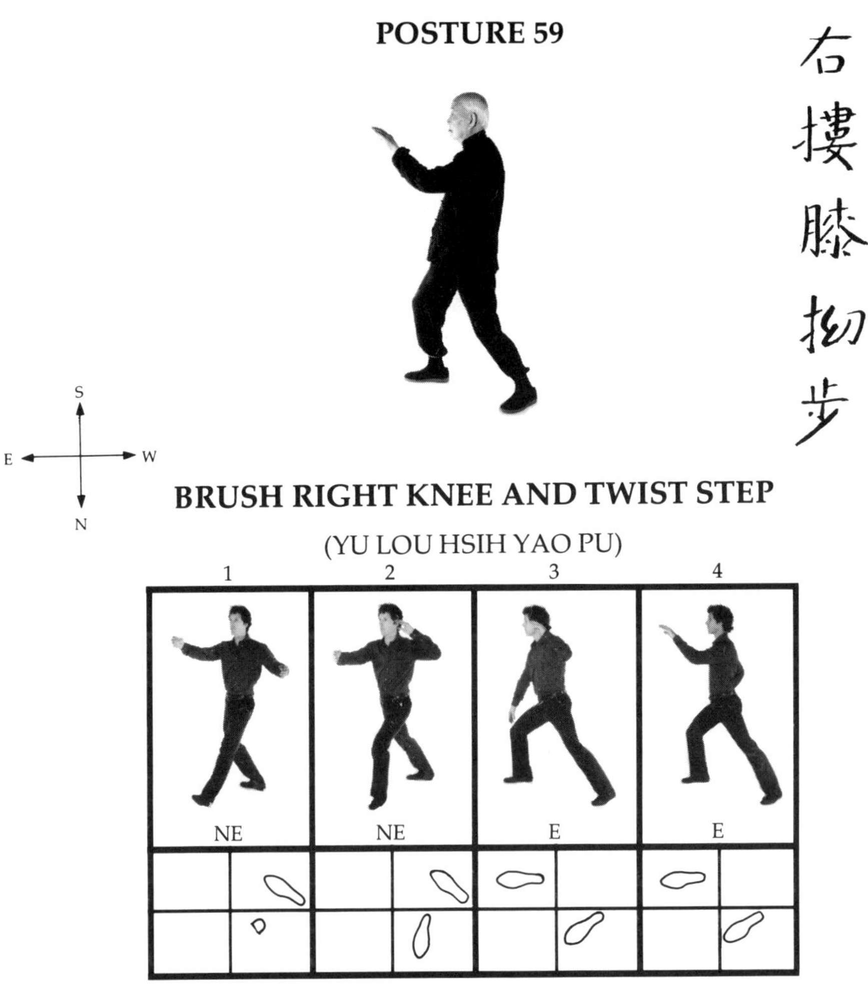

This posture is the same as posture #15.

POSTURE 60

進步栽捶

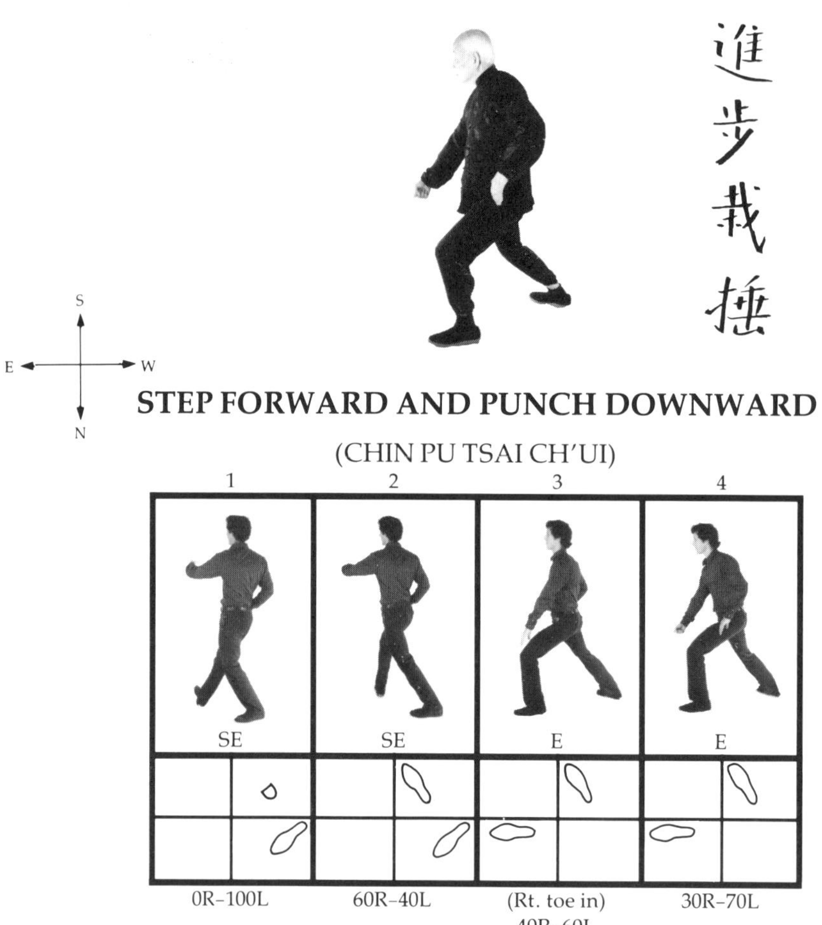

STEP FORWARD AND PUNCH DOWNWARD

(CHIN PU TSAI CH'UI)

During the Counts of:

1. Withdraw your weight to the left foot and turn the torso slightly to the right, turning the right foot slightly outward to point southeast.
2. Make a fist with your right hand and hold the "tiger mouth" (space between thumb and forefinger) upward, by your right thigh. The left arm is bent and is chest height with the palm facing the body. Shift your weight to your right foot.
3. Take a step directly forward with your left foot, heel touching first, and shift the weight to it. Brush your left knee with your left hand and hold it beside the thigh (palm backward), and turn your right foot slightly inward (pivoting on the heel).
4. Shift 70% of your weight to the left foot and punch downward with your right fist below and near your left knee with the "tiger mouth" facing forward. You are still facing east.

POSTURE 61

轉身撇身捶

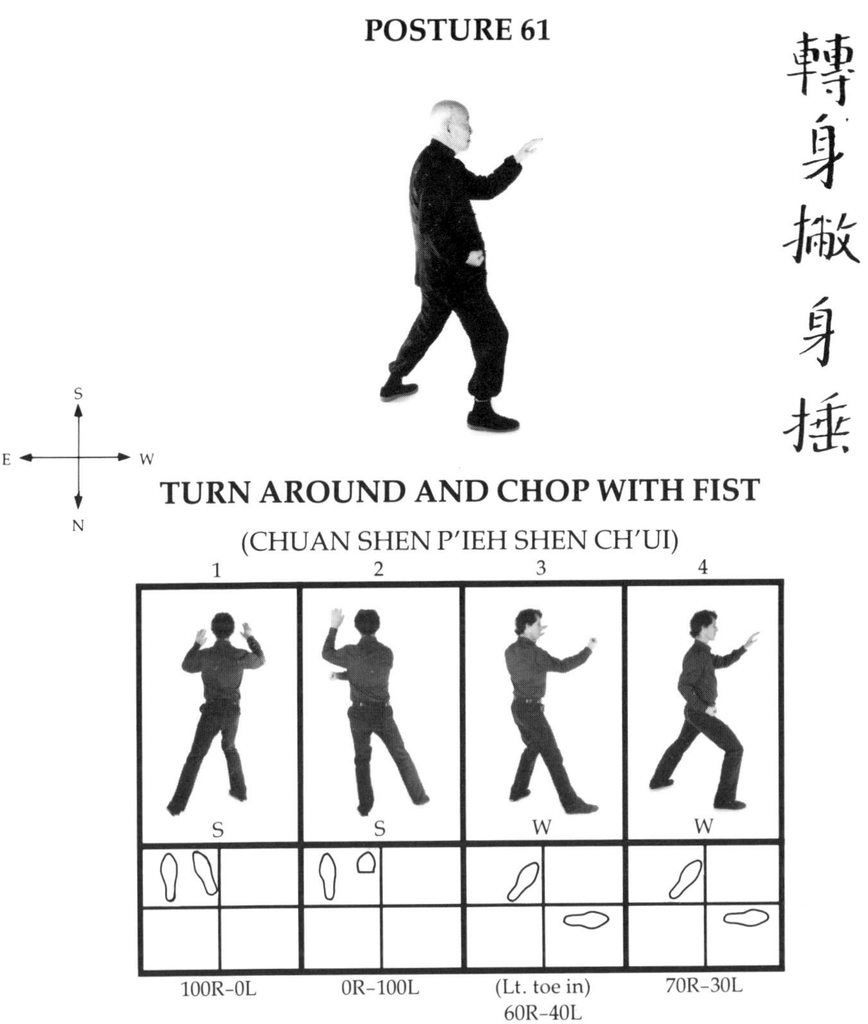

TURN AROUND AND CHOP WITH FIST

(CHUAN SHEN P'IEH SHEN CH'UI)

During the Counts of:

1. Open your right fist and immediately begin circling both your hands clockwise (upward, and rightward) while turning your body to the right (south) and shifting your weight to the right foot. At the same time turn your left foot inward so that it points south.
2. Continue to circle your hands clockwise (downward, leftward and upward) until your let hand is near your left temple, with the palm outward and elbow bent. Your right circles to the front of your left chest clenched in a fist with the knuckles upward. At the same time shift your weight to the left foot and let the right heel rise slightly.
3. Turn your body to the right (west). Raise your right foot and take a half step in the forward right direction with the heel touching first and toes pointing west. Make your right fist circle upward to the right and chop downward toward the west; withdraw it to the right side of your waist with the knuckles down. The left hand circles down to a position in front of the left chest, palm

outward. At the same time slowly shift your weight to your right foot and turn your left foot slightly inward. (Note: The picture for this count does not show the movement at the end of the count. The picture enables the learner to see the actual "chop").

4. Shift 70% of your weight to your right foot and push forward with your left palm from its position in front of your chest. You are now facing west.

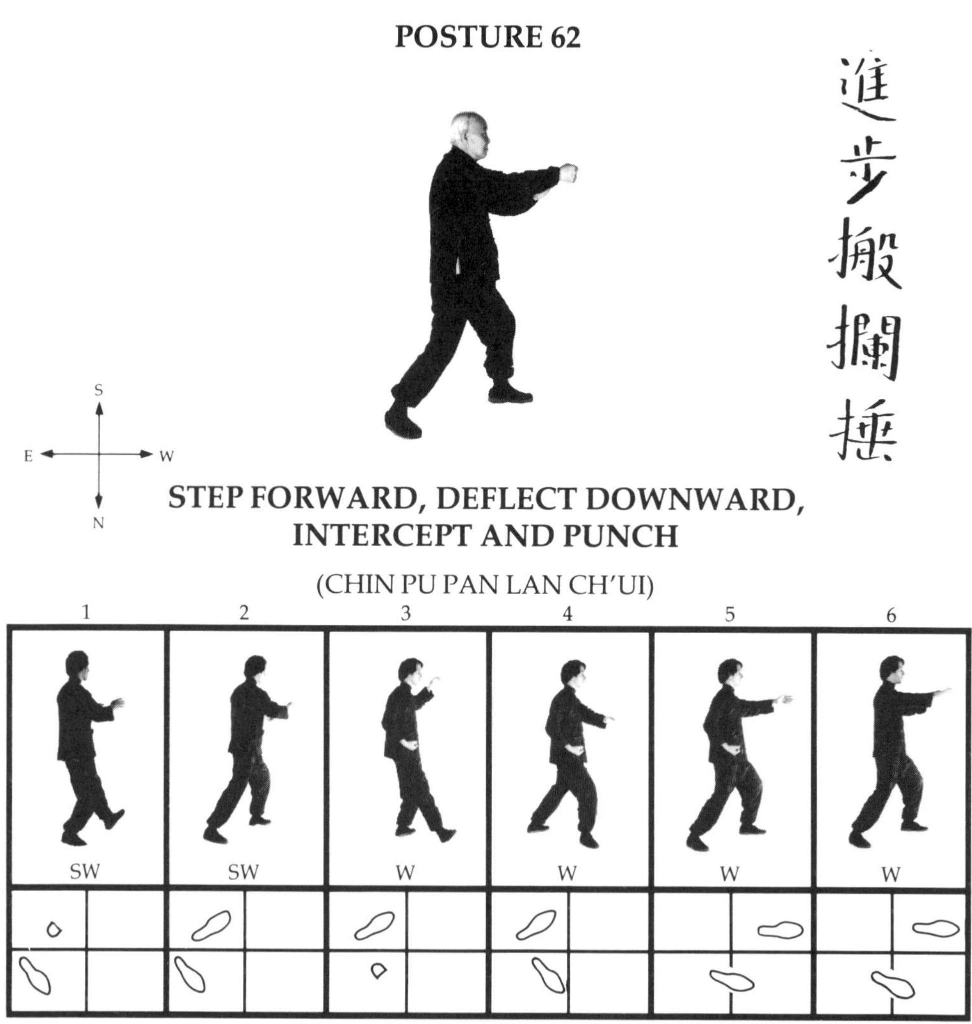

POSTURE 62

STEP FORWARD, DEFLECT DOWNWARD, INTERCEPT AND PUNCH

(CHIN PU PAN LAN CH'UI)

This posture is the same as posture #20.

POSTURE 63

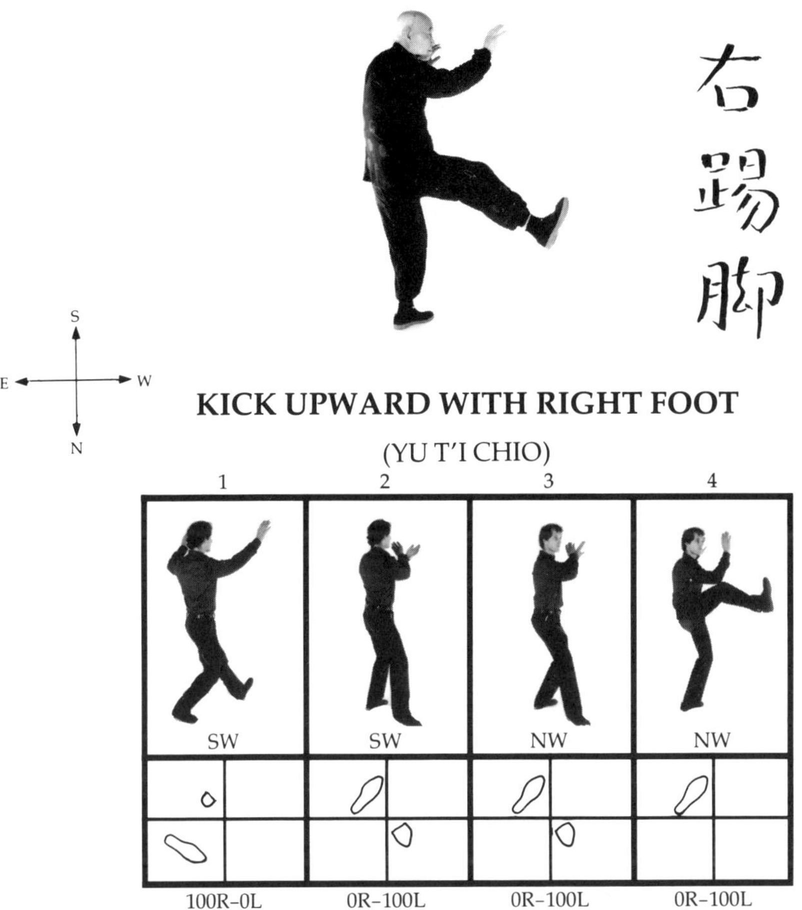

KICK UPWARD WITH RIGHT FOOT

(YU T'I CHIO)

During the Counts of:

1. Draw your body backward and shift your weight to your right foot. Turn the left toes slightly outward and turn your body slightly to the left (to face SW). At the same time open your right fist, separate your hands and start to circle them in opposite directions (upward and outward — right hand clockwise, left hand counterclockwise).
2. Shift the weight forward to your left foot. At the same time continue to circle your hands downward and inward. As they approach each other along the lower arc of the circle bring them upward and cross them diagonally at the wrists in front of your left foot. The right foot slides to the front (W) one half-step with only the toes touching the ground, pointing northwest.
3. Turn the palms outward and turn your body slightly to the right (to face NW).
4. Kick upward as high as you can comfortably with the tip of your right foot, the sole facing NW. At the same time chop forward with your right hand at the level of your nose, while your left arm is bent behind and to the left of the left ear. The fingers of the left hand point upwards, so as to maintain balance. You are now facing NW.

POSTURE 64

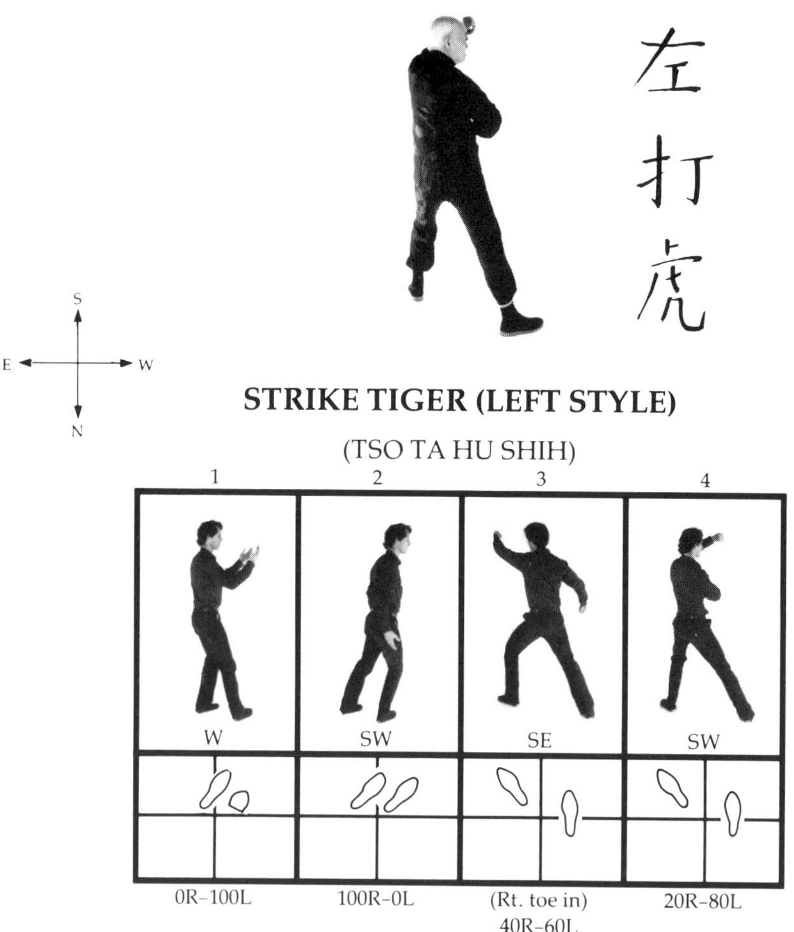

STRIKE TIGER (LEFT STYLE)

(TSO TA HU SHIH)

During the Counts of:

1. Lower your right foot and put it down in front and to the right of your left foot. Circle your right hand clockwise, with the palm upward and lower the arm so that it is chest level. The left hand is lowered from its position by the ear so that the arm is parallel to the right arm. Both elbows are bent. You are facing west.
2. Shift the weight to the right leg. Continue to circle your right hand, downward to the waist level, with the palm upward, and continue to circle your left hand clockwise downward in front of your chest with the palm downward. You are facing SW.
3. Gradually turn your body to the SE and take a big step diagonally in this direction with your left foot (heel touching first) and gradually shift your weight to it. Pivot the right foot slightly inward. At the same time clench both hands into fists and continue to circle your right hand leftward at about waist level while your left hand continues to circle clockwise — downward, leftward and upward.

4. Shift 80% of your weight to the left leg with the knee bent. Continue to circle your hands until your right fist is at the left side of your waist with knuckles upward and your left fist is above your left forehead with knuckles inward. You are now facing SW.

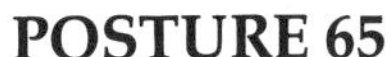

POSTURE 65

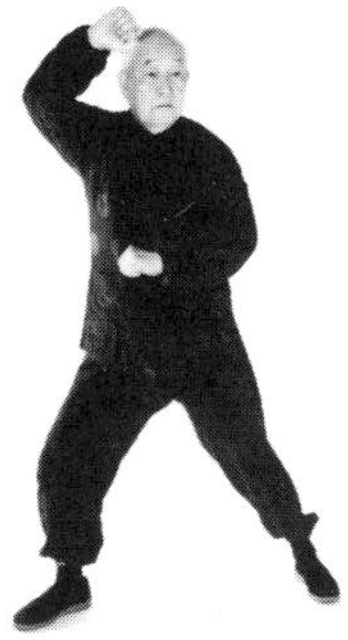

右打虎

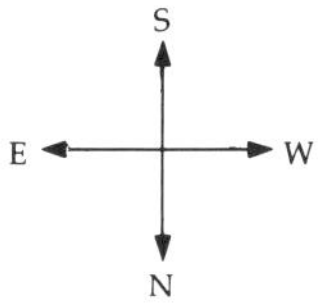

S
E W
N

STRIKE TIGER (RIGHT STYLE)

(YU TA HU SHIH)

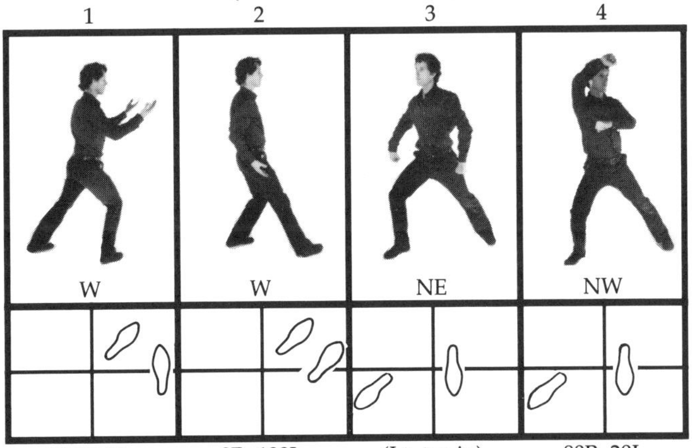

1	2	3	4
W	W	NE	NW
100R–0L	0R–100L	(Lt. toe in) 60R–40L	80R–20L

During the Counts of:

1. Turn your body to the right (west) and shift your weight to the right foot and curve your left toes inward as much as you can. Both arms circle forward, palms up and out from the chest.
2. Continue to lower your arms in front of your lower abdomen. Shift the weight to your left foot. The right foot pivots on the toe to point southwest.
3. (The same as posture #64, except where indicated). Step NE and face NE. The right fist moves counterclockwise to the right and up and the left fist clockwise to the left and up.
4. Right fist above, left below. Turn the waist to face NW.

POSTURE 66

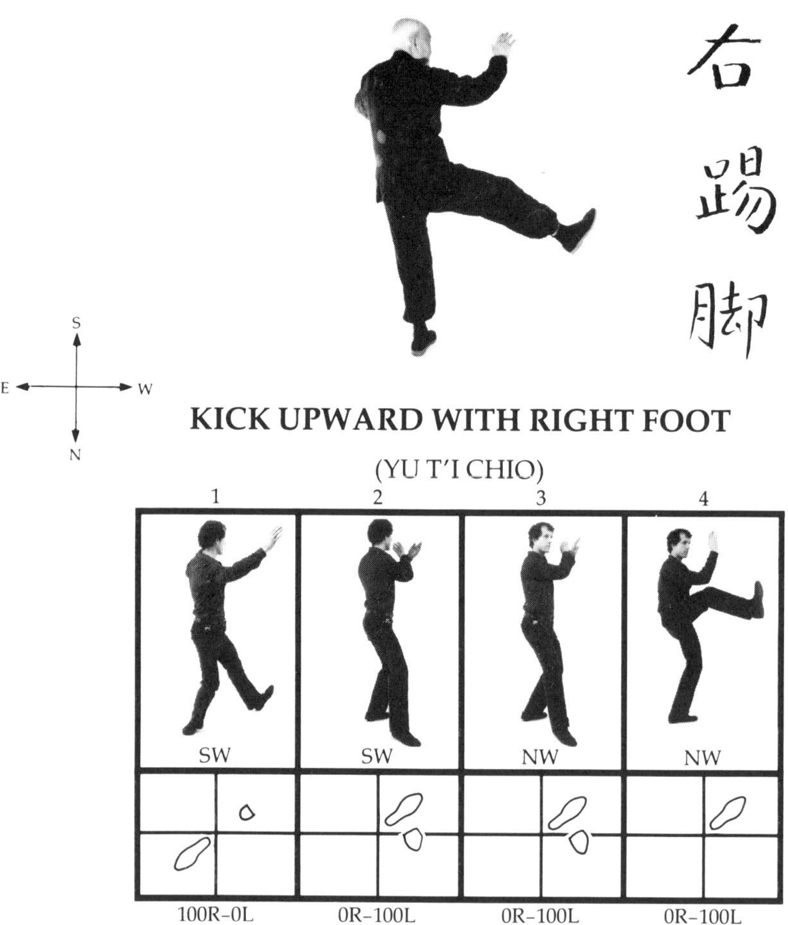

KICK UPWARD WITH RIGHT FOOT

(YU T'I CHIO)

During the Counts of:

1. Turn your body to the left (southwest). Turn the left foot outward by pivoting on the heel and turn your right foot slightly inward. At the same time open the fists and start to circle the hands upward and sideways in opposite directions. The right arm circles rightward and the left, leftward.
2. Shift your weight to the left foot and bring your right foot in front of your left foot, with the toes touching the ground. Continue to circle your hands in opposite directions, downward and then upward in front of you, crossing them at your chest (wrists join together). The palms face inward and the right hand is placed inside of the left hand.
3. Turn your body to the right (northwest). At the same time turn your palms outward.
4. Kick upward with the tip of your right foot, the sole facing toward the northwest. Your right hand chops forward in the same direction to ear level with the fingers pointing upward and your left hand, with the fingers pointing up, is held behind by your left ear to maintain balance. You are now facing northwest.

POSTURE 67

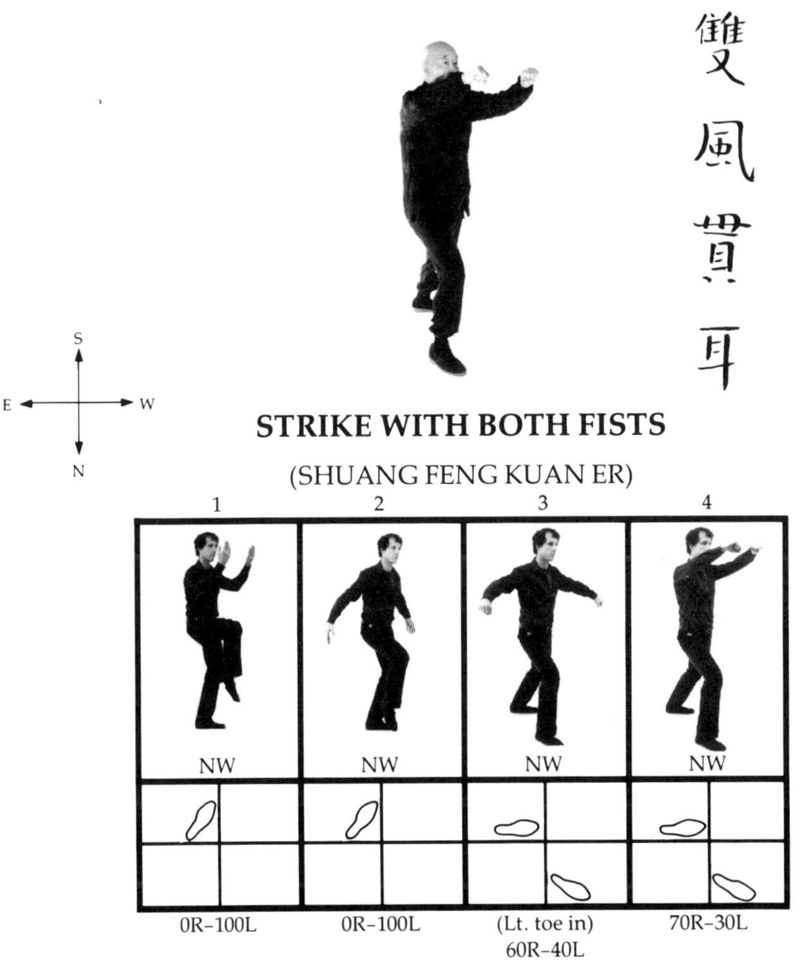

STRIKE WITH BOTH FISTS

(SHUANG FENG KUAN ER)

During the Counts of:

1. Lower and suspend your right foot with the toes pointing down, bending the knee and keeping the thigh level.
2. Lower your hands with palms upward and brush the two sides of your suspended right knee.
3. Step forward and rightward with your right foot (heel touching first, toes pointing northwest) and gradually shift weight to it. Turn your left foot slightly inward. At the same time clench your hands into fists and begin to circle them backward and upward.
4. Shift 70% of your weight to the right foot. Continue to circle your fists upward and strike forward and inward, stopping them in front of your head with the knuckles upward (tiger mouths facing each other). The elbows are slightly bent (the fists are about shoulder width apart). You are still facing northwest.

POSTURE 68

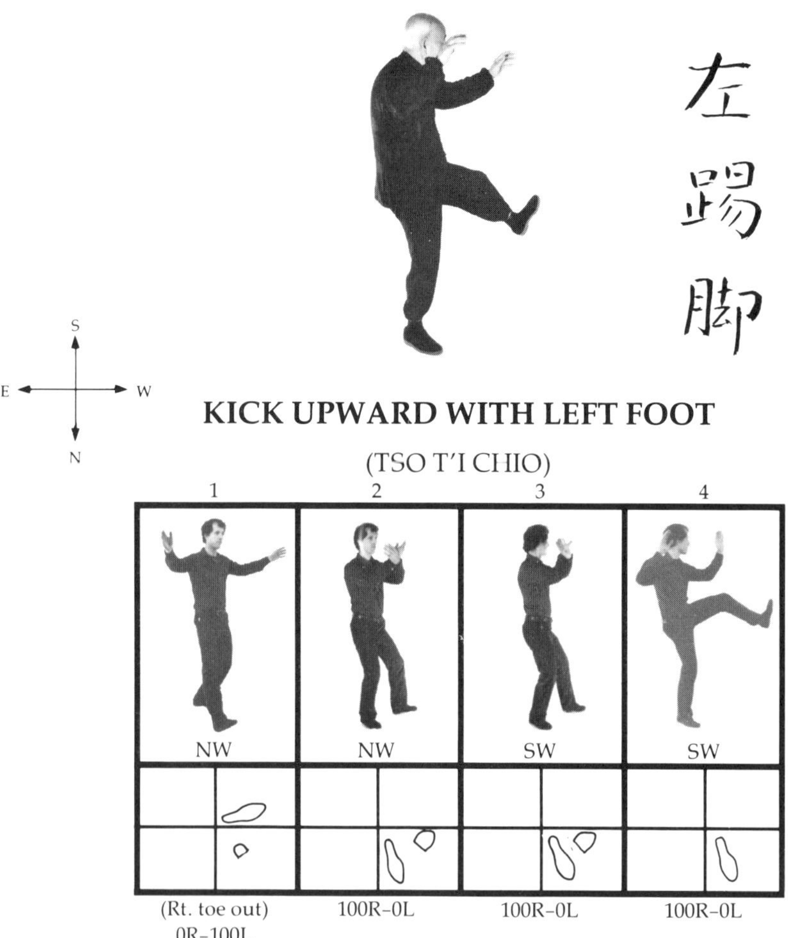

KICK UPWARD WITH LEFT FOOT

(TSO T'I CHIO)

During the Counts of:

1. Shift the weight to your left foot and turn your right foot slightly outward. Open the fists and circle the hands down to the sides in opposite directions, the right hand moving rightward and the left hand, leftward.
2. Shift the weight to your right foot. Withdraw your left foot and put it beside and slightly in front of your right foot with only the toes touching the ground pointing southwest. Continue to circle your hands downward and inward, and cross them at the wrists in front of your chest. The right hand is outside of the left hand and the palms face inward.
3. Turn the palms outward. At the same time turn your body to the left (southwest).
4. Kick upward with the tip of your left foot with the sole facing southwest. At the same time chop forward with your left hand at the level of your ear; your right arm is bent with the hand behind and by the right ear with fingers pointing upward so as to maintain balance. You are now facing southwest.

POSTURE 69

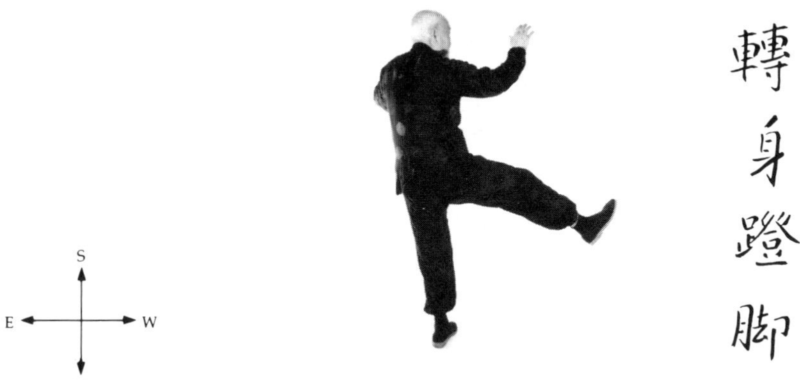

TURN AROUND AND KICK WITH SOLE (RIGHT FOOT)

(CHUAN SHEN TENG CHIO)

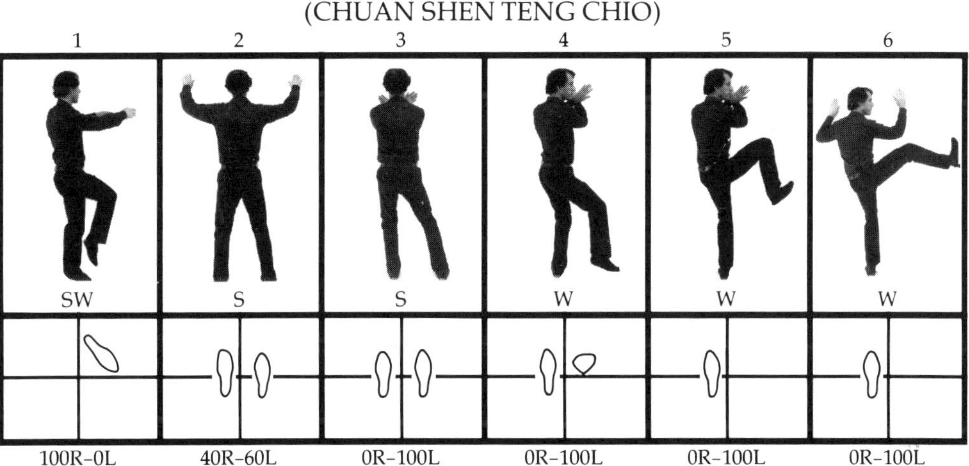

During the Counts of:

1. Lower your left hand sideways to the level of your chest and withdraw your left foot, bending the knee with the foot suspended in the air and toes pointing down. At the same time turn the leg slightly to the left, lower the right hand and bring it toward the left in line with the left arm.
2. Raise your right heel and turn your body around to the far right by pivoting on the ball of the right foot, until you face south. Lower your left foot to the ground with the toes pointing south and begin to shift the weight to it.
3. Circle your hands in opposite directions, upward, outward, sideways and downward, as you shift all the weight to the left leg.
4. Continue to circle your hands, inward and upward, and cross them in front of your chest, with wrists joined and the right hand placed inside of the left hand (palms facing inward). Shift your right foot slightly backward in front of your left foot, with only the toes touching the ground, pointing southwest.
5. Turn your palms outward and gradually turn your torso to the right (west). Raise your right thigh with the knee bent and toes slightly upward.

6. Kick forward (west) with your right sole, with toes upward, while you chop forward with your right hand at the level of your nose. Your left arm is bent back behind your left ear with the fingers pointing upward so as to maintain balance. Now you are facing west.

POSTURE 70

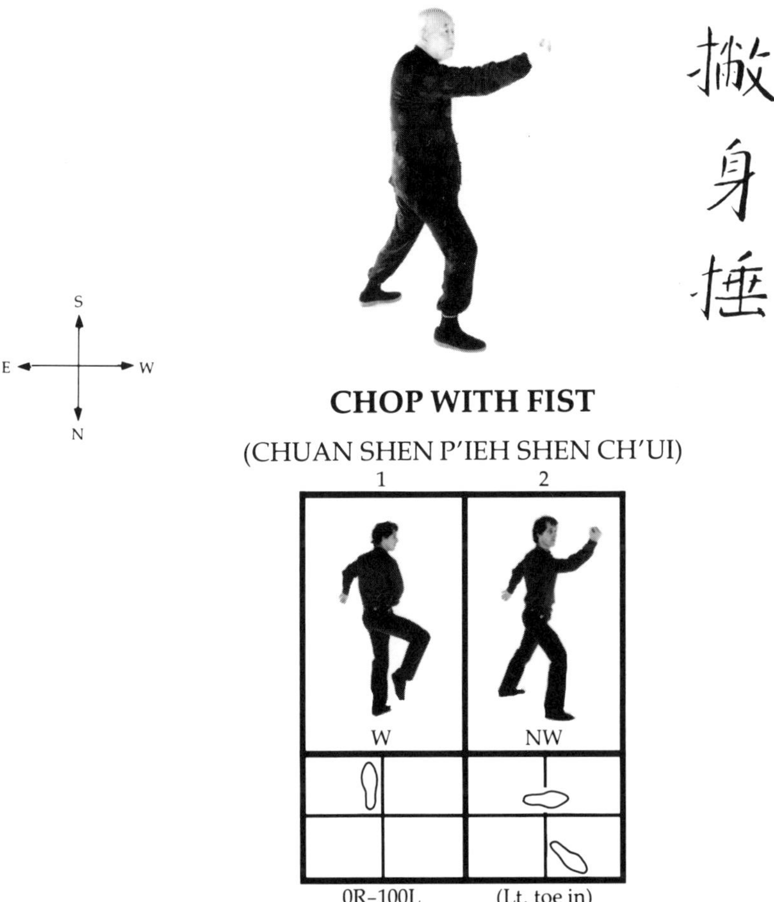

CHOP WITH FIST

(CHUAN SHEN P'IEH SHEN CH'UI)

During the Counts of:

1. Draw back and suspend your right foot with the knee bent and toes pointing down. Circle your right hand clockwise, downward and leftward, with the palm inward; lower your left hand with the palm outward.
2. Clench your right hand into a fist and shift your right foot diagonally to the right. Put it down, with heel touching first and toes pointing northwest, and gradually shift 70% of your weight to it. Turn your left foot slightly inward. At the same time continue to circle your right fist upward on the left, and chop rightward at head level with the knuckles down. Simultaneously extend your left hand behind you at the level of your waist, with the palm down and fingers pointing southeast. Your eyes are looking at the right fist. You are now facing northwest.

POSTURE 71

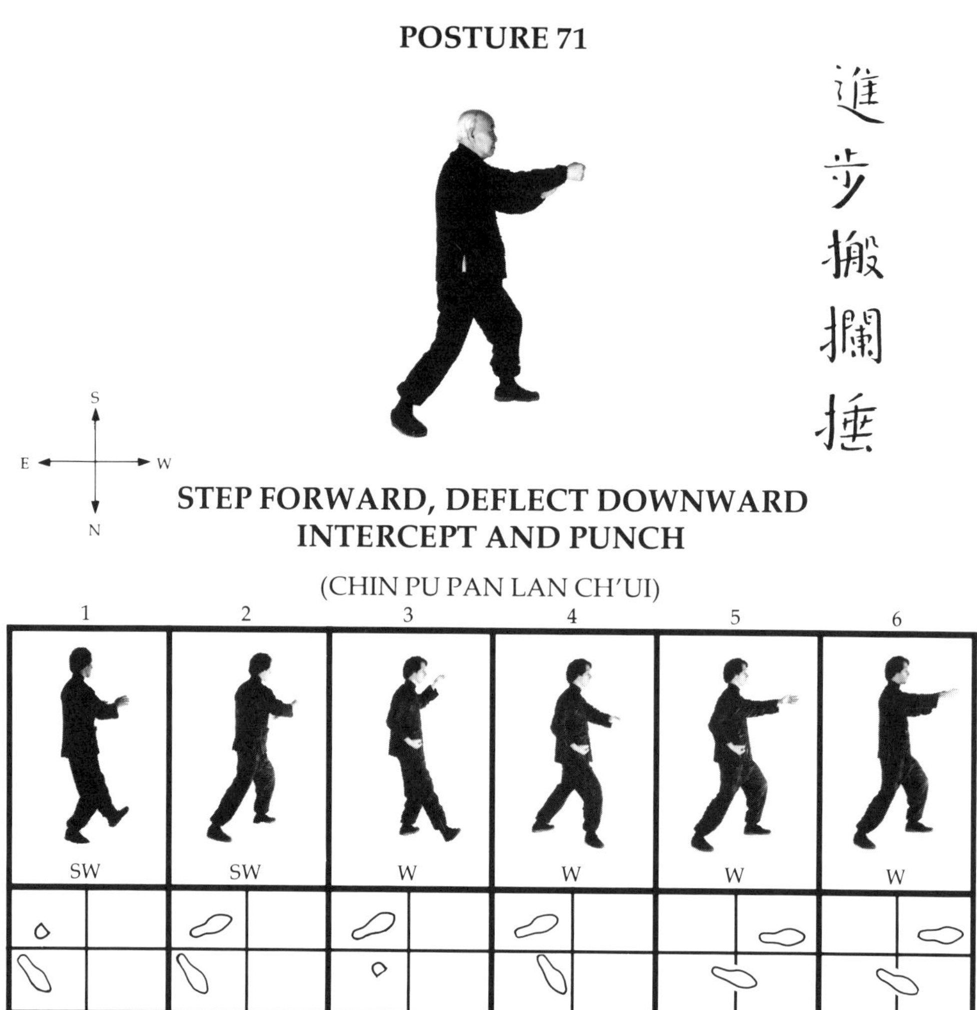

STEP FORWARD, DEFLECT DOWNWARD INTERCEPT AND PUNCH

(CHIN PU PAN LAN CH'UI)

During the Counts of:

1. Pick up your left foot and set it down turned slightly outward in the SW direction.

Beats 2 to 6 are the same as the respective beats of posture #20.

POSTURE 72

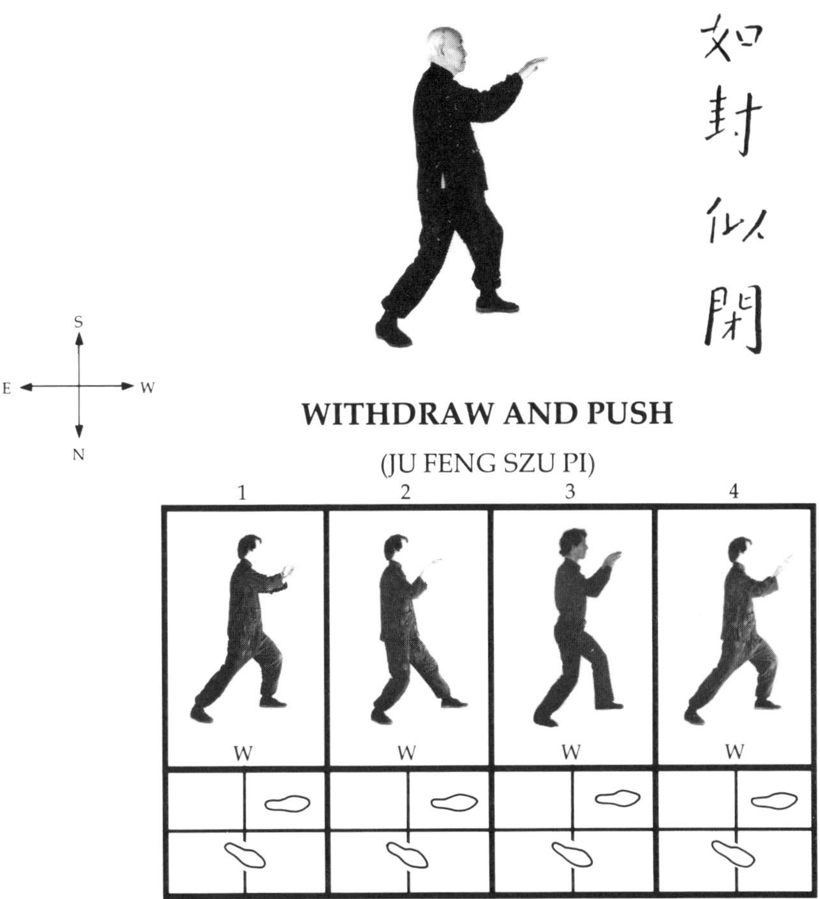

WITHDRAW AND PUSH

(JU FENG SZU PI)

This posture is the same as posture #21.

POSTURE 73

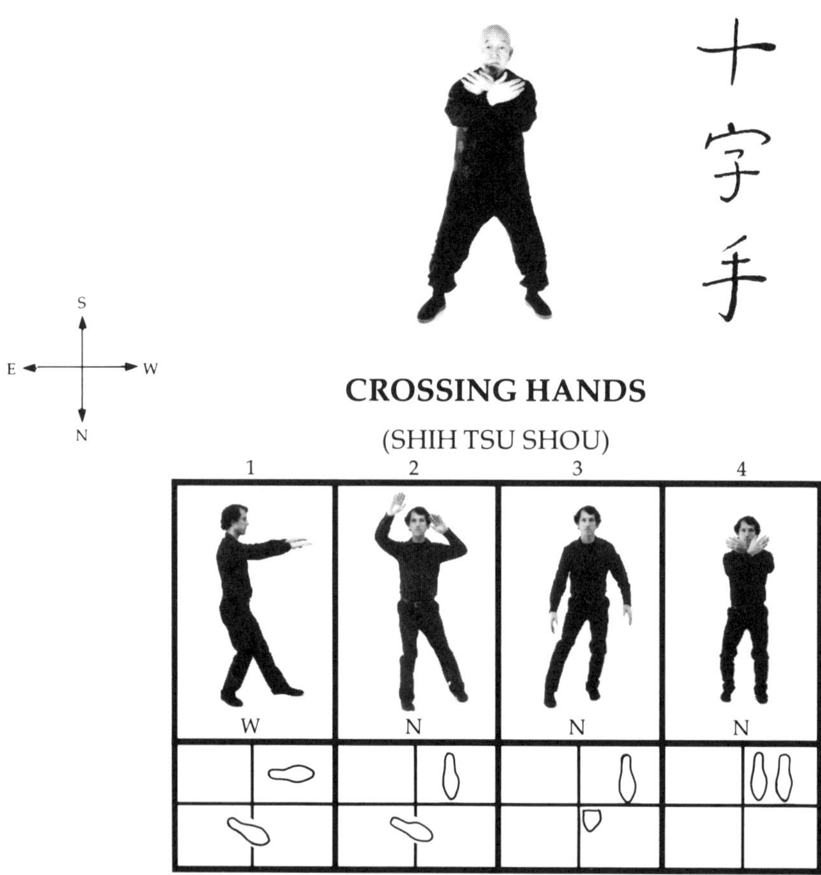

CROSSING HANDS

(SHIH TSU SHOU)

This posture is the same as posture #22.

POSTURE 74

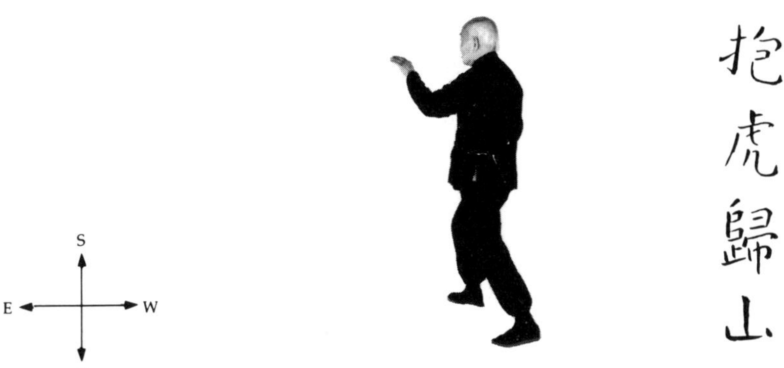

EMBRACE THE TIGER AND RETURN TO THE MOUNTAIN

(PAO HU KUEI SHAN)

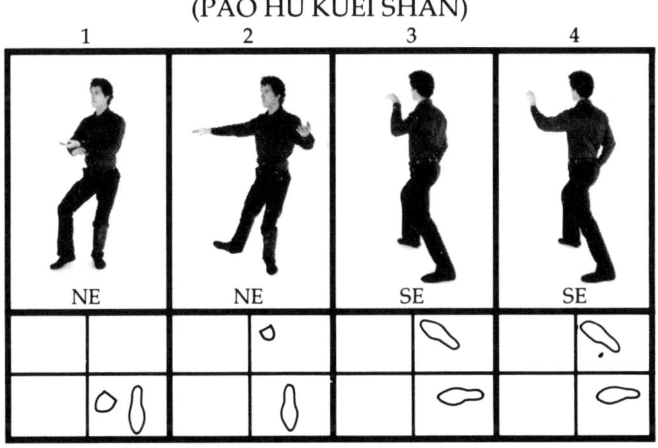

This posture is the same as posture #23.

POSTURE 75

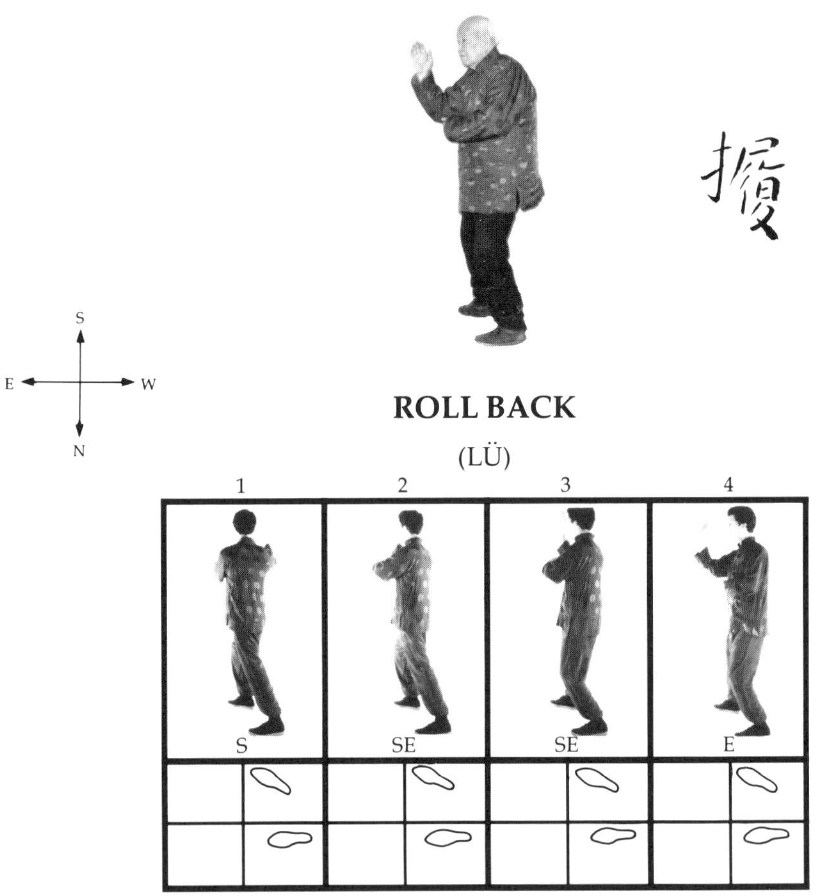

ROLL BACK

(LÜ)

This posture is the same as posture #5.

POSTURE 76

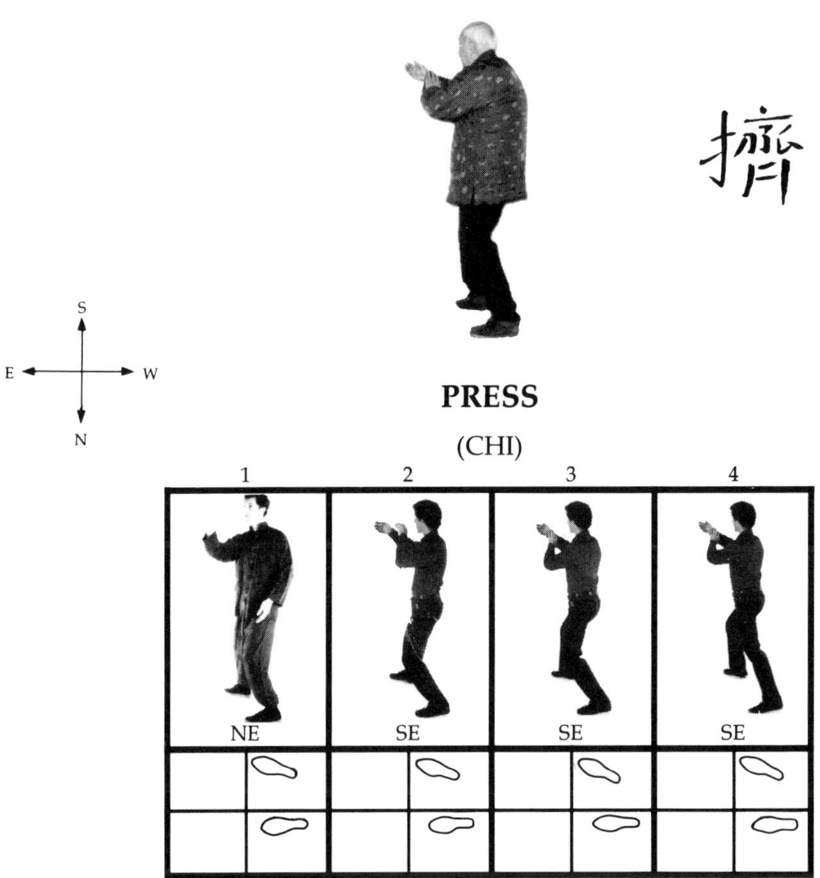

This posture is the same as posture #6.

POSTURE 77

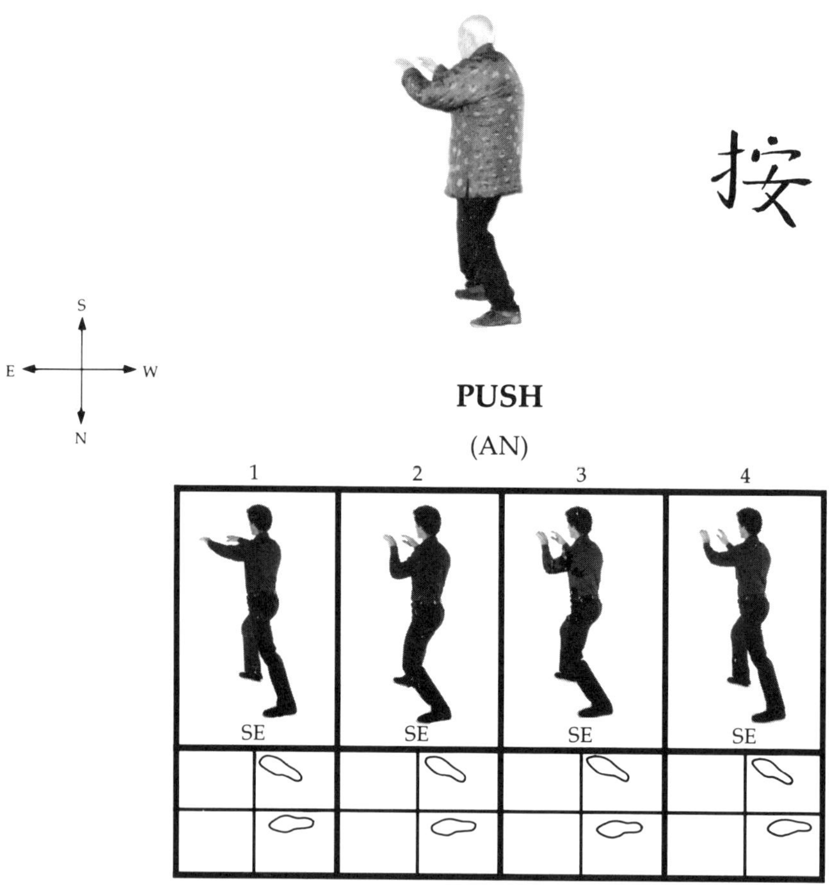

PUSH

(AN)

This posture is the same as posture #7.

POSTURE 78

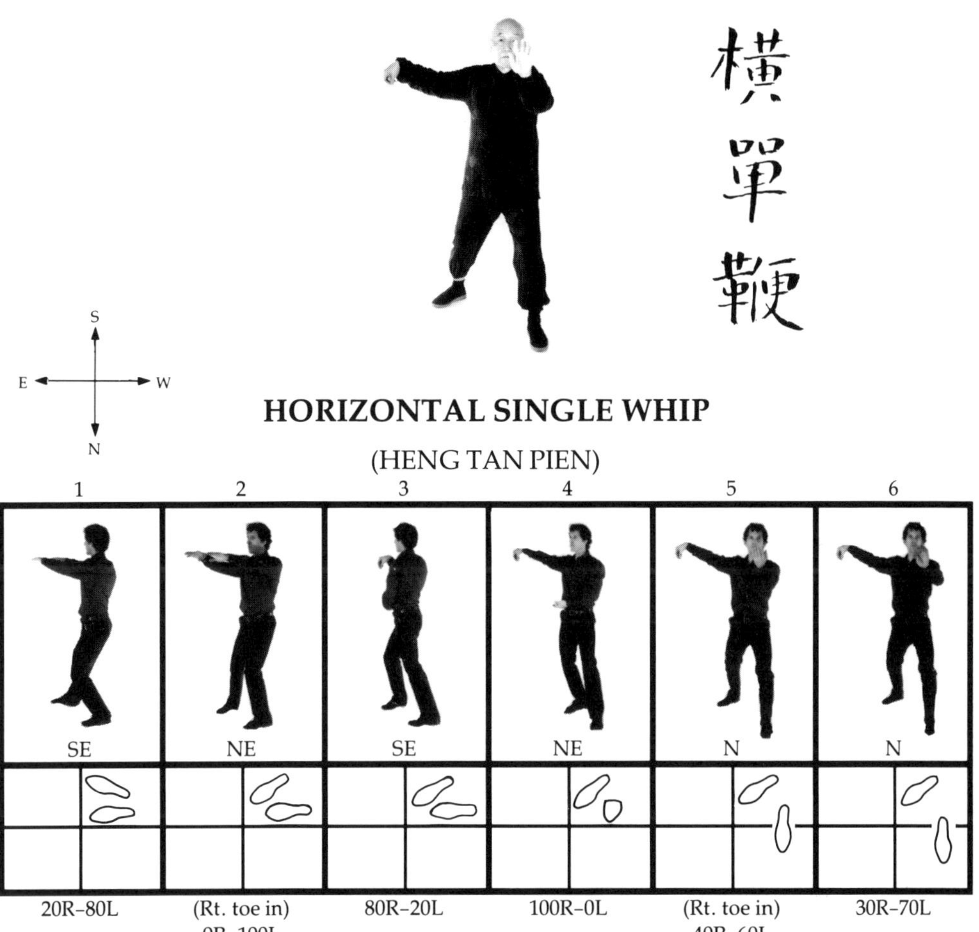

HORIZONTAL SINGLE WHIP

(HENG TAN PIEN)

During the Counts of:

1. Shift your weight gradually to your left foot; your palms face downward; your hands are parallel with your shoulders.
2. Turn your torso to the left until it faces northeast. At the same time pivot on your right heel, carrying the toes slightly inward.
3. As you shift your weight back to your right leg, allow the body to turn to the right so that you face southeast. As you bend your right elbow to withdraw your right hand southward, allow the fingers to point down and lightly close together at the tips (as if holding a drop of water) thus forming a hook near the right armpit. Bring the left hand to rest, palm up, under the right breast.
4. Pivot on the ball of the left foot, so that the toes point northeast with the rising heel turning rightward. Extend the ''hook hand'' rightward so that the knuckles face southeast. The trunk turns NE.
5. As your trunk continues to turn leftward, step to the front left (north) with your left foot, heel down first and then toes (to point north). The left heel

should not be directly in front of your right heel. The feet should be in as wide a diagonal position as you can manage comfortably. Gradually shift your weight to your left foot (bending the left knee) and allow your waist to turn left ward so that you face north; the left hand with the palm turning inward, is carried leftward until it is opposite the left breast and at the same time raise your right foot slightly and turn it slightly inward by pivoting on the heel.

6. Continue to shift your weight to the left foot until 70% of your weight has been shifted to it. Turn your left palm outward with the arm slightly bent, as your eyes, which have accompanied the gradual turn, look past the finger tips. You are now facing north.

POSTURE 79

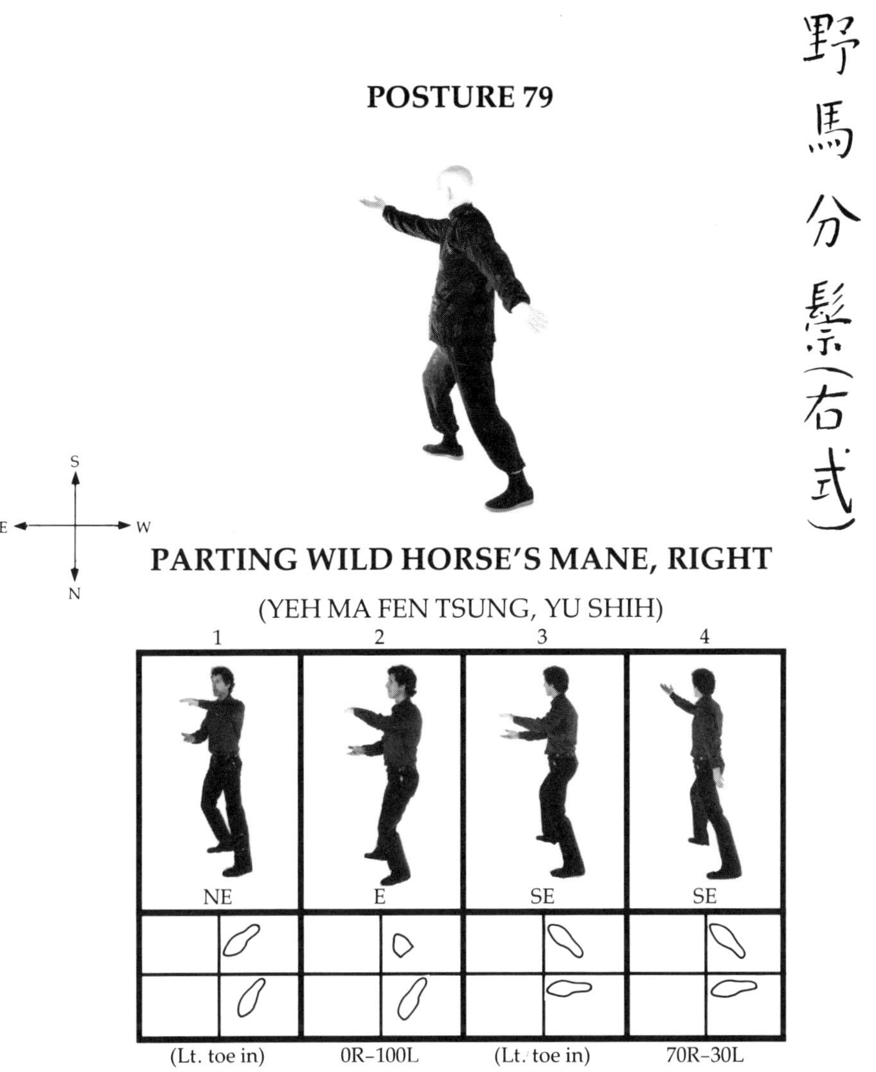

PARTING WILD HORSE'S MANE, RIGHT

(YEH MA FEN TSUNG, YU SHIH)

During the Counts of:

1. Shift your weight to the right foot, turn your body to the right (northeast) and turn your left foot slightly inward.
2. Shift your weight to the left foot. Continue to turn your body to the right (to face east) until the right foot is brought to its toes, pointing southeast. At the same time bring your left hand over toward your throat, with the palm down and elbow bent. Open your right "hook hand" and lower it near your left waist with the palm up, you simulate holding a ball in your hands.
3. Take a half-step forward with your right foot toward the southeast (heel touching first) and shift the weight to it. Turn the left foot slightly inward. Continue to turn your body to the right (southeast) and at the same time begin to gradually raise your right forearm forward toward the southeast, and slantingly upward. During this move your left hand downward.
4. Shift 70% of your weight to the right foot and continue to raise your right forearm until your right hand is at the height of your nose with palm facing

slanting upward over your right leg and fingers pointing southeast. Move your left hand downward and backward until it is angled behind your left thigh with the palm facing southwest. You are now facing southeast.

POSTURE 80

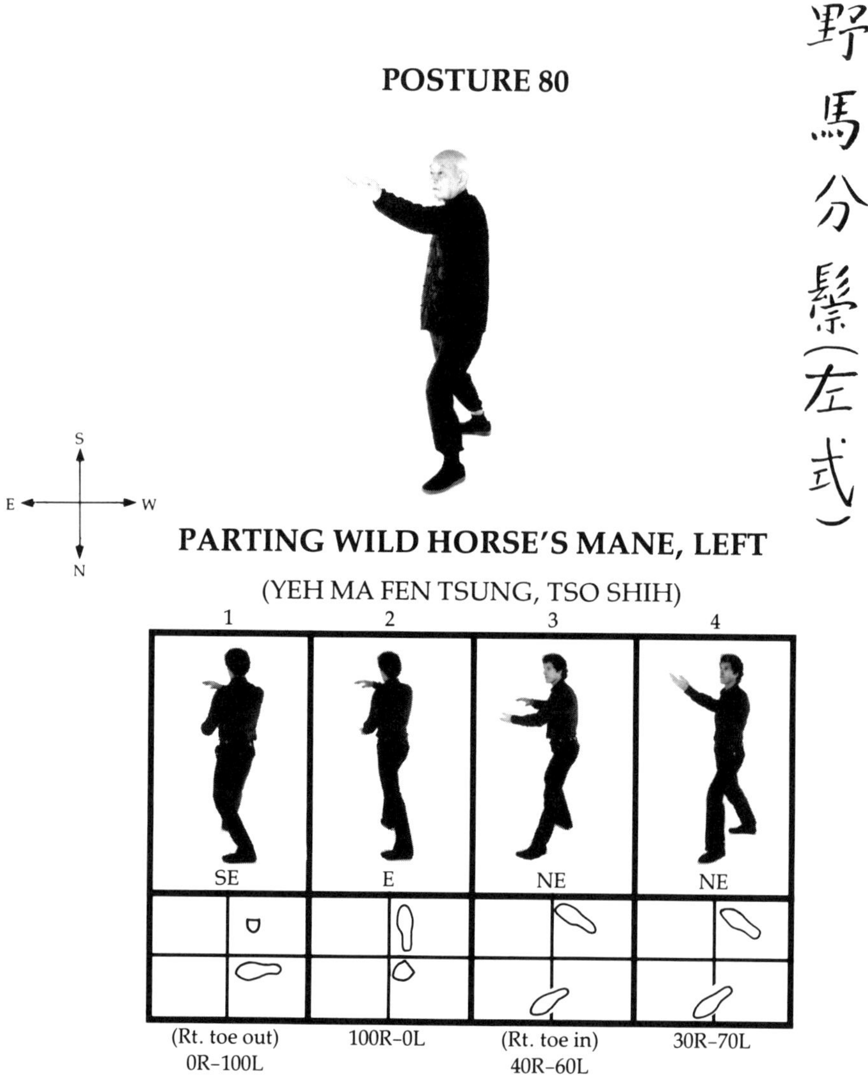

PARTING WILD HORSE'S MANE, LEFT

(YEH MA FEN TSUNG, TSO SHIH)

During the Counts of:

1. Shift your weight to the left foot and turn your right foot slightly outward on the heel.
2. Shift your weight to the right foot and lower your right hand to the height of your throat with palm down, elbow bent, and move your left hand near the right side of your waist with the palm upward. You simulate holding a ball in your hands. Turn your body gradually to the left (to face east).
3. Take a half-step forward (northeast) with your left foot, heel touching first, and shift the weight to it; curve the right foot slightly inward. At the same time begin to gradually raise your left forearm forward and slantingly upward

and move your right hand downward. (Note: photograph three of this posture does not show the completion of the count, only the left foot stepping.)

4. Shift 70% of your weight to the left foot. Continue to raise your left forearm forward (toward the northeast) and slantingly upward until it is at the height of your nose with the palm facing upward at an angle over your left leg. The fingers of the left hand point northeast. At the same time move your right hand downward and backward until it stops behind your right thigh with the palm facing northwest. You are now facing northeast.

POSTURE 81

PARTING WILD HORSE'S MANE, RIGHT

(YEH MA FEN TSUNG, YU SHIH)

野馬分鬃(右式)

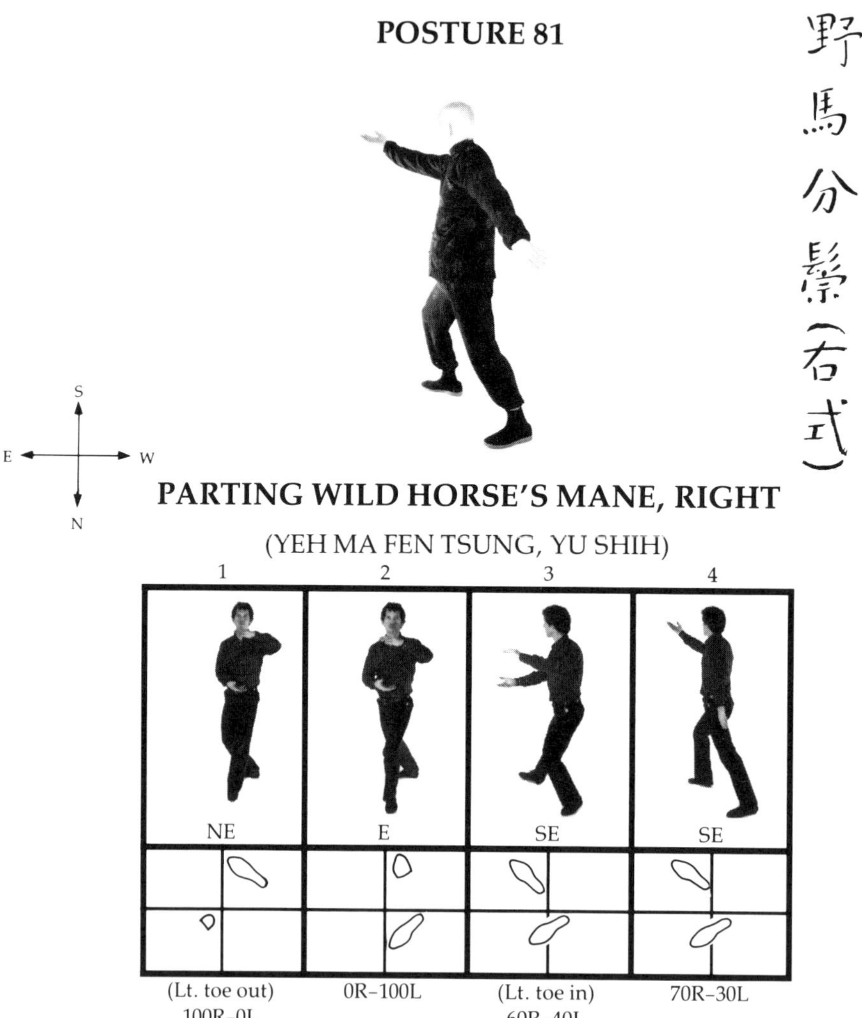

During the Counts of:

1. Shift your weight to your right foot and turn your left foot slightly outward.
2. Shift your weight to your left foot and turn your body gradually to the right (to face NE) so that the right foot is raised up onto its toes. Lower your left hand near your throat with palm down, elbow bent, and move your right hand near your left waist with palm up. Again you simulate holding a ball in your hands.
3. Take a half-step forward with your right foot toward the southeast (heel touching first) and gradually shift the weight to it. Turn the left foot slightly inward. Continue to turn your body to the right (southeast). At the same time begin to gradually raise your right forearm forward and slantingly upward and move your left hand downward. (Note: photograph three of this posture does not show the completion of the count, only the left foot stepping.)
4. Shift 70% of your weight to the right foot. Continue to raise your right forearm forward (toward the southeast) and slantingly upward until it is at the height of your nose, with the palm facing upward over your right leg and the fingers pointing southeast. Move your left hand downward and backward where it stops behind your left thigh with the palm facing southwest. You are now facing southeast.

POSTURE 82

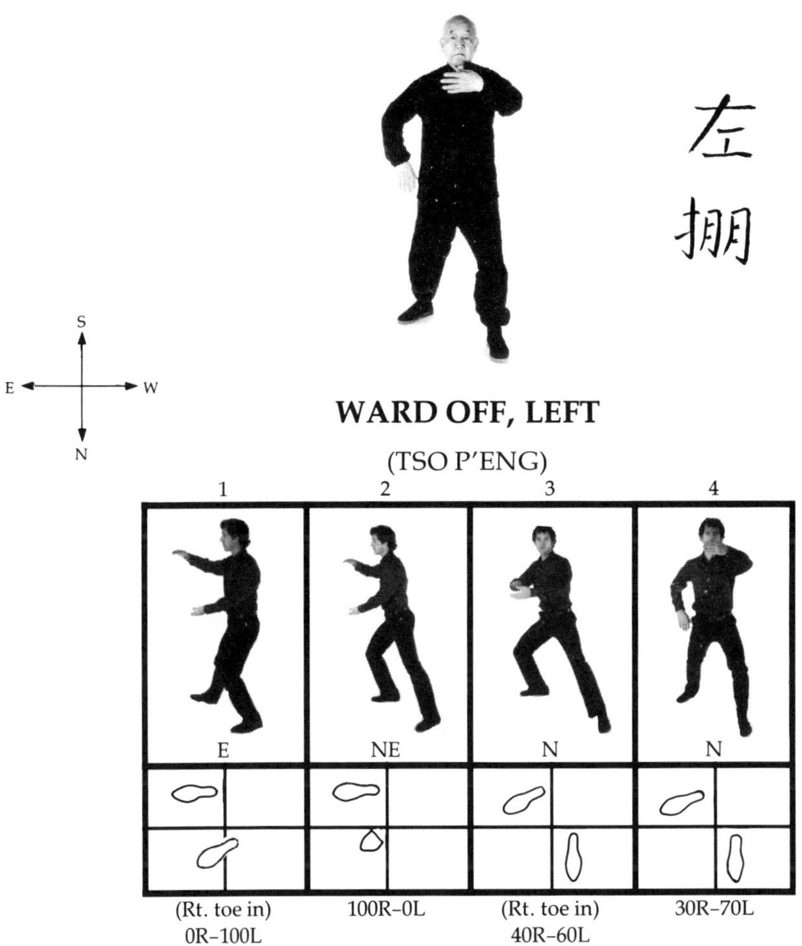

WARD OFF, LEFT

(TSO P'ENG)

During the Counts of:

1. Shift your weight back to your left foot and turn your right foot slightly inward. At the same time withdraw and lower your right hand near your throat with the palm down and move your left hand near the right side of your waist with the palm up. You simulate holding a ball in your hands and turn your body slightly to the left (east).
2. Shift your entire weight to the right foot and continue to turn your body slightly to the left (to face northeast) so that the left foot is raised up onto its toes.
3. Touching first with the heel, place the left foot slightly leftward (toward the north) and gradually shift the weight onto it. Continue to turn the upper torso to the left (to face north) and at the same time raise the left arm, (elbow slightly down) while lowering the right arm. Pivoting on the heel, turn the right foot slightly inward so that the toes point northeast. (Note: This picture does not show the beat at its completion. It shows the step forward only).

4. Shift 70% of the weight to your left foot. Continue to raise the left arm until the palm of the hand faces the chest and continue to lower the right arm until the hand rests beside the right hip joint, with the palm backward. The eyes have accompanied the turning movement and now look directly ahead (north). You are facing north.

POSTURE 83

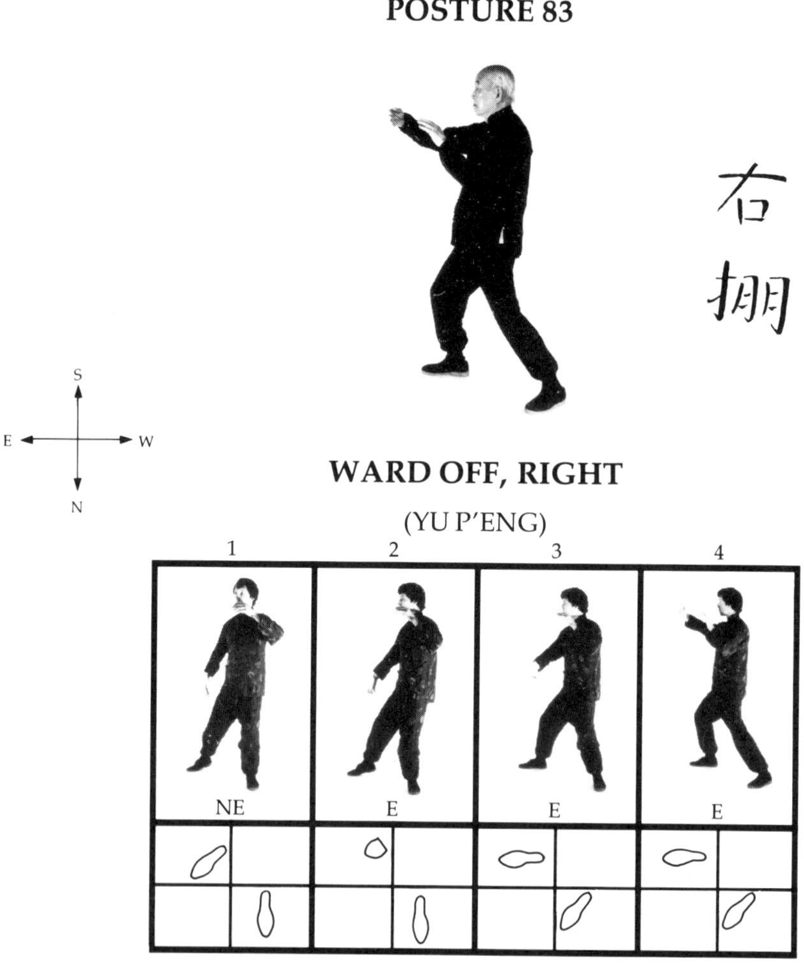

WARD OFF, RIGHT

(YU P'ENG)

This posture is the same as posture #4.

POSTURE 84

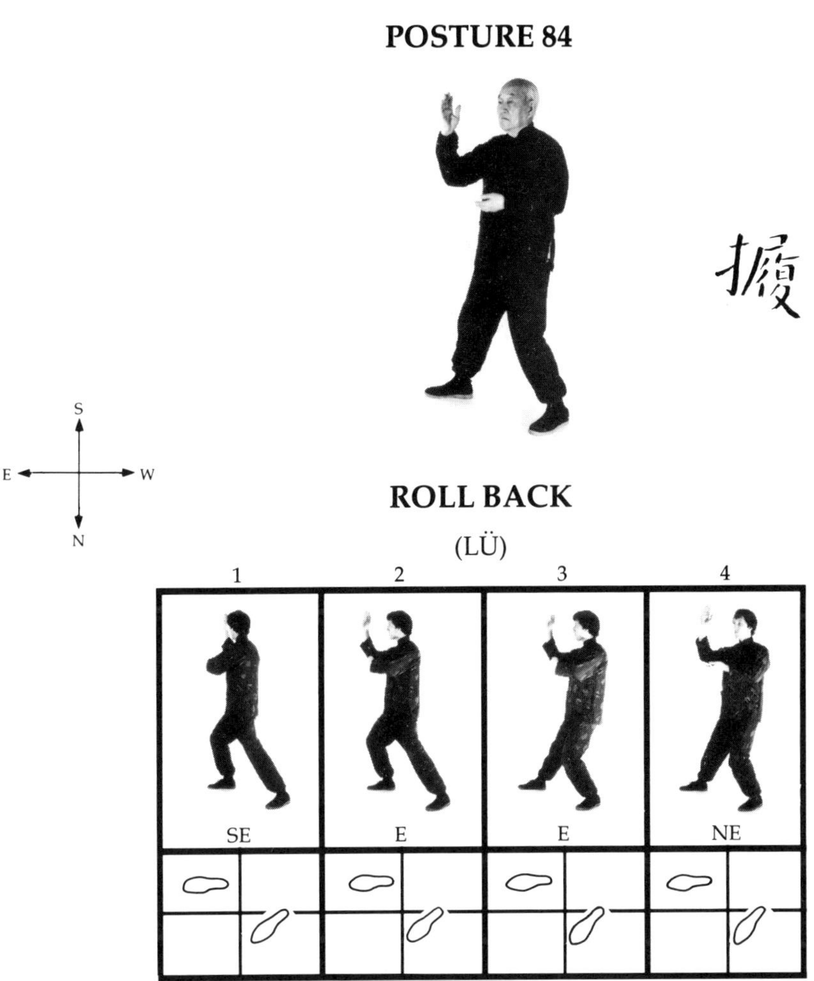

ROLL BACK

(LÜ)

This posture is the same as posture #5.

POSTURE 85

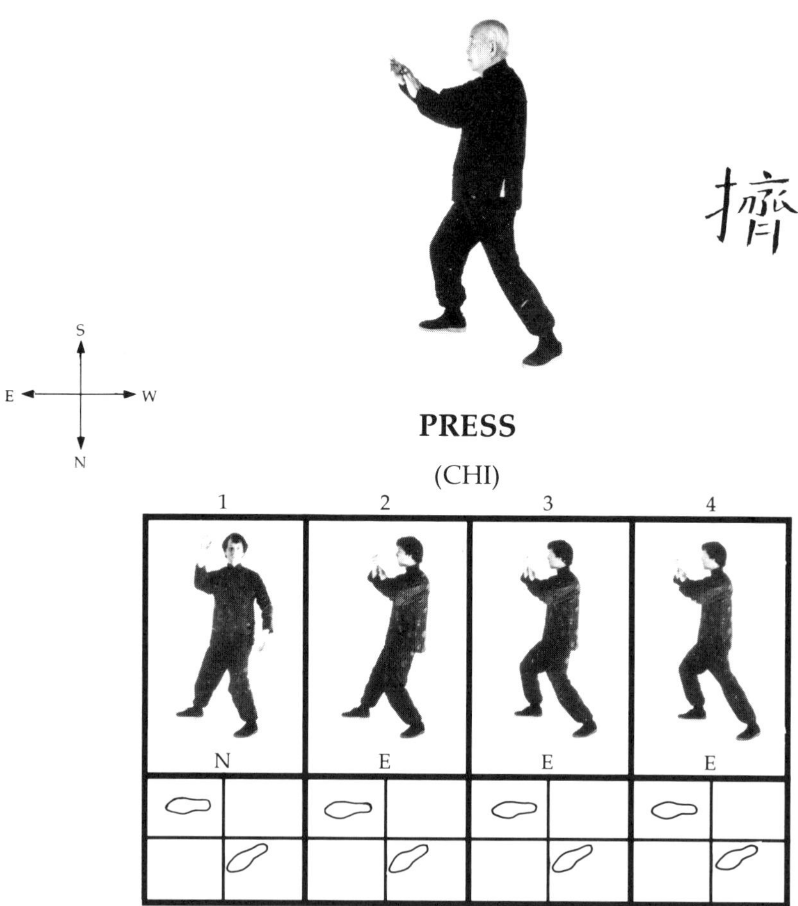

PRESS

(CHI)

This posture is the same as posture #6.

POSTURE 86

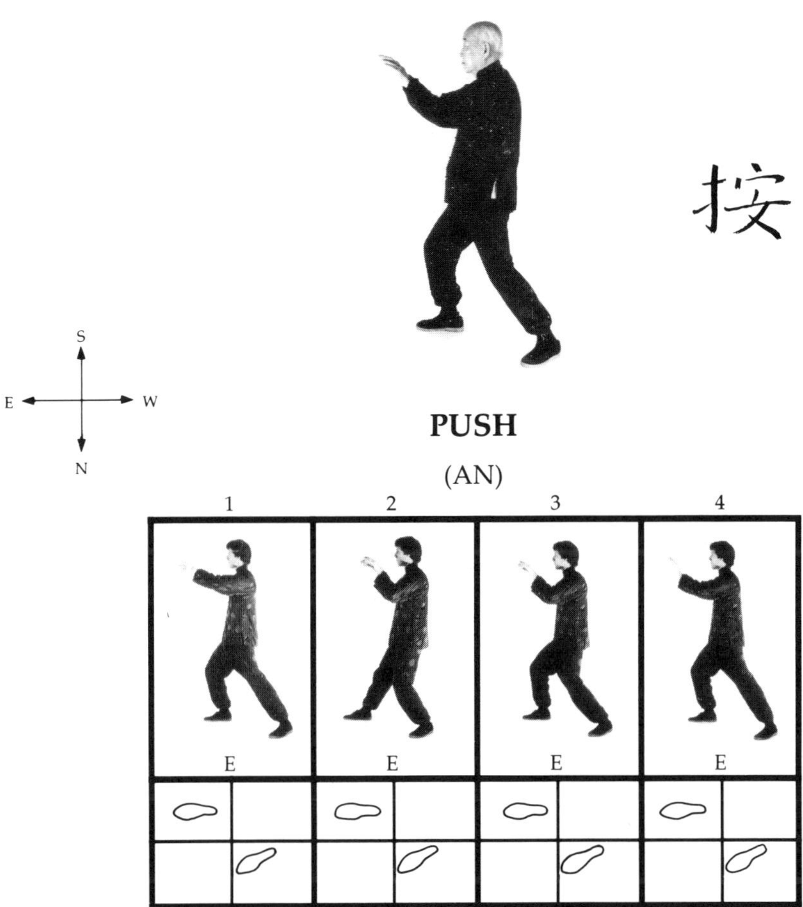

PUSH

(AN)

This posture is the same as posture #7.

POSTURE 87

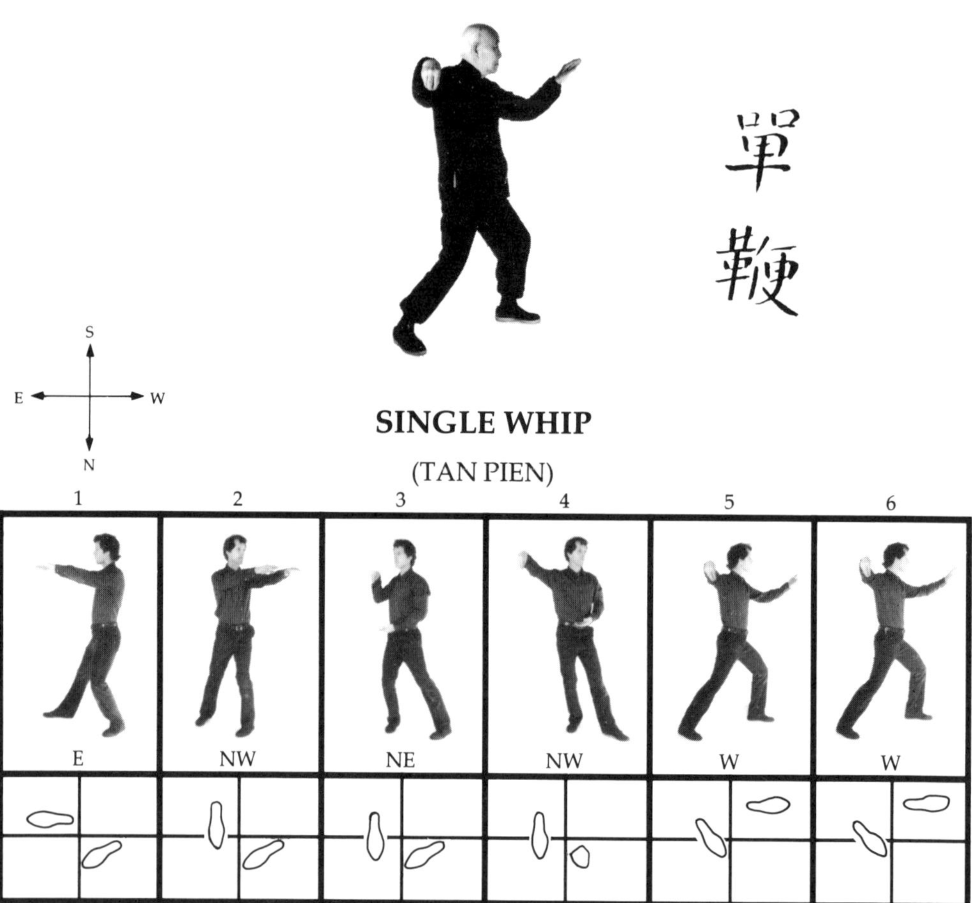

This posture is the same as posture #8.

POSTURE 88

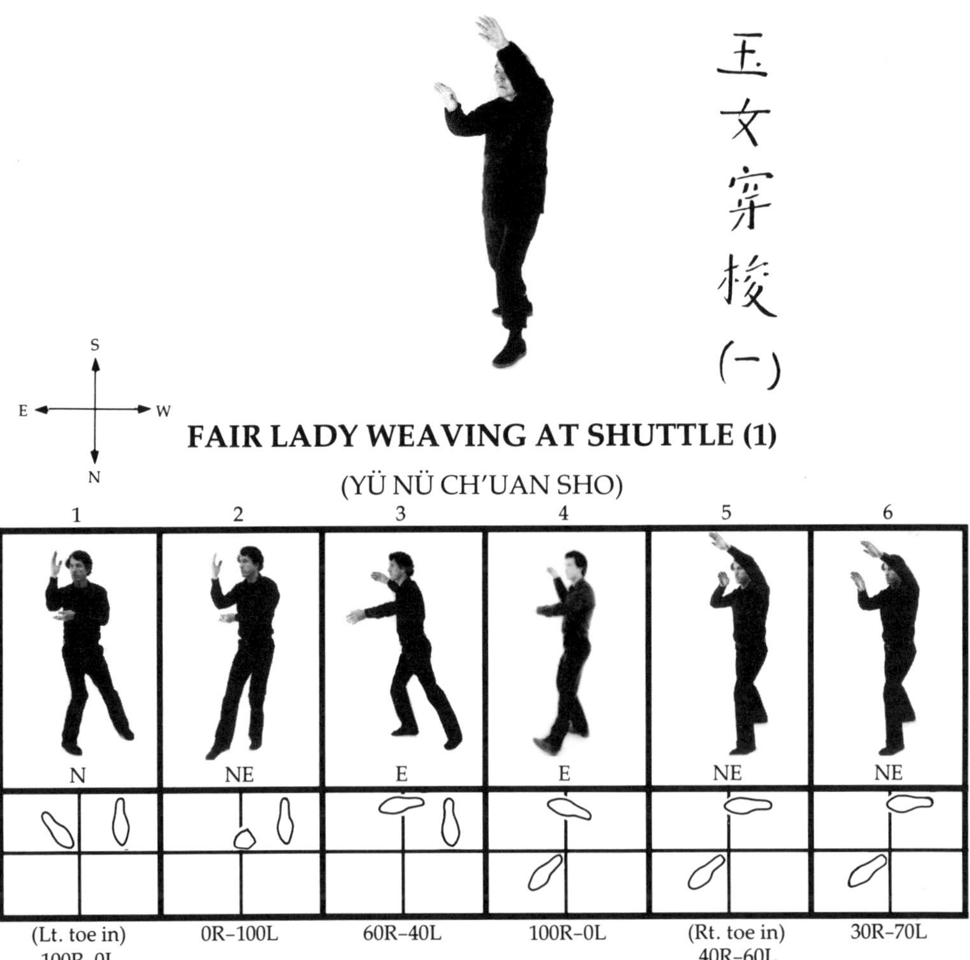

FAIR LADY WEAVING AT SHUTTLE (1)

(YÜ NÜ CH'UAN SHO)

During the Counts of:

1. Shift your weight to the right foot. Gradually turn your body to the right (to face north) and pivoting on the left heel, turn the left foot inward so that the toes point north. At the same time draw back your left hand near your right waist with the palm upward and opening your right "hook hand", bring it near your right ear with the palm down and elbow bent.
2. Shift your weight to the left foot so that the right foot is brought onto its toes (pointing northeast), and continue to turn your body to the right (to face northeast).
3. Shift your right foot slightly to the forward right direction with the heel touching first and toes pointing southeast set it down. Continue to turn your body to the right (to face east) and gradually shift the weight to the right foot. At the same time raise your left hand, palm inward, toward its upper left, and circle your right hand counterclockwise downward and backward.
4. Take a step with your left foot forward to the northeast, heel touching first,

continue to circle your right hand upward and forward, stop it near your right ear with palm forward and elbow bent.

5. Continue to raise your left hand upward until it is over your left forehead and turn the palm outward. The right hand moves, palm outward, to the front of the body. At the same time gradually turn your body to the left (to face northeast), and begin to shift your weight to the left foot; turn your right foot slightly inward.
6. Shift 70% of your weight to the left foot and push your right hand forward (with the energy of the whole body) with the right elbow slightly bent, keeping the palm outward. You are now facing northeast.

POSTURE 89

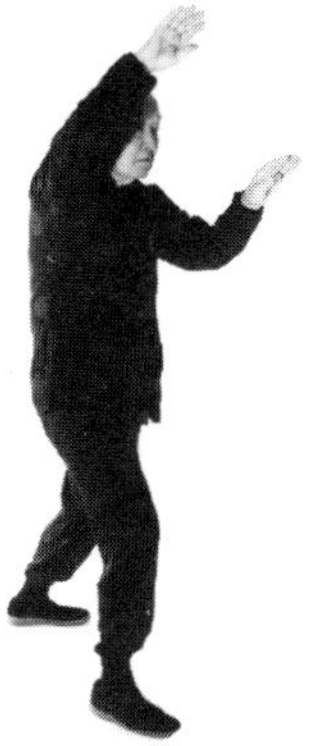

玉女穿梭(二)

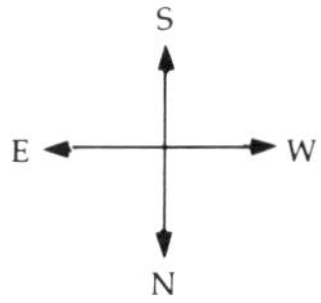

S / E / W / N

FAIR LADY WEAVING AT SHUTTLE (2)

(YÜ NÜ CH'UAN SHO)

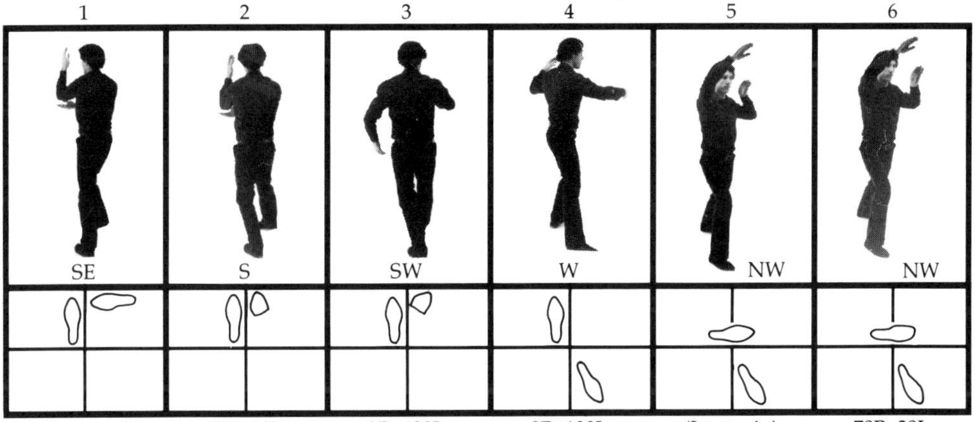

1	2	3	4	5	6
SE	S	SW	W	NW	NW
(Lt. toe in) 100R-0L	0R-100L	0R-100L	0R-100L	(Lt. toe in) 60R-40L	70R-30L

During the Counts of:

1. Shift your weight to your right foot and slowly turn your body to the right (to face SE) while pivoting on the left heel. Turn the left foot inward as far as possible so that the toes point south. At the same time lower your right hand near your left waist, with the palm upward, and bend your left arm so that the left hand with the palm inward and fingers pointing upward is near your left ear.
2. Shift your weight to the left foot so that the right foot is brought to its toes pointing southwest. At the same time continue to turn your body gradually to the right (to face south).
3. Raise your right hand rightward and upward with the palm inward and circle your left hand clockwise downward and backward, while continuing to turn your body to the right (to face SW).
4. Take a step northwest with your right foot with the heel touching first and toes pointing northwest. At the same time continue to circle your left hand,

upward and forward to stop near your left ear with the elbow bent and palm forward.

5. Gradually shift your weight to the right foot and continue to turn your body to the right (to face northwest). At the same time raise your right hand over your forehead with the palm forward and elbow bent. Turn your left foot slightly inward. The left hand moves to the front of the body.
6. Shift 70% of your weight to the right foot and push forward with your left hand together with the energy of your whole body as one unit. You are now facing northwest.

POSTURE 90

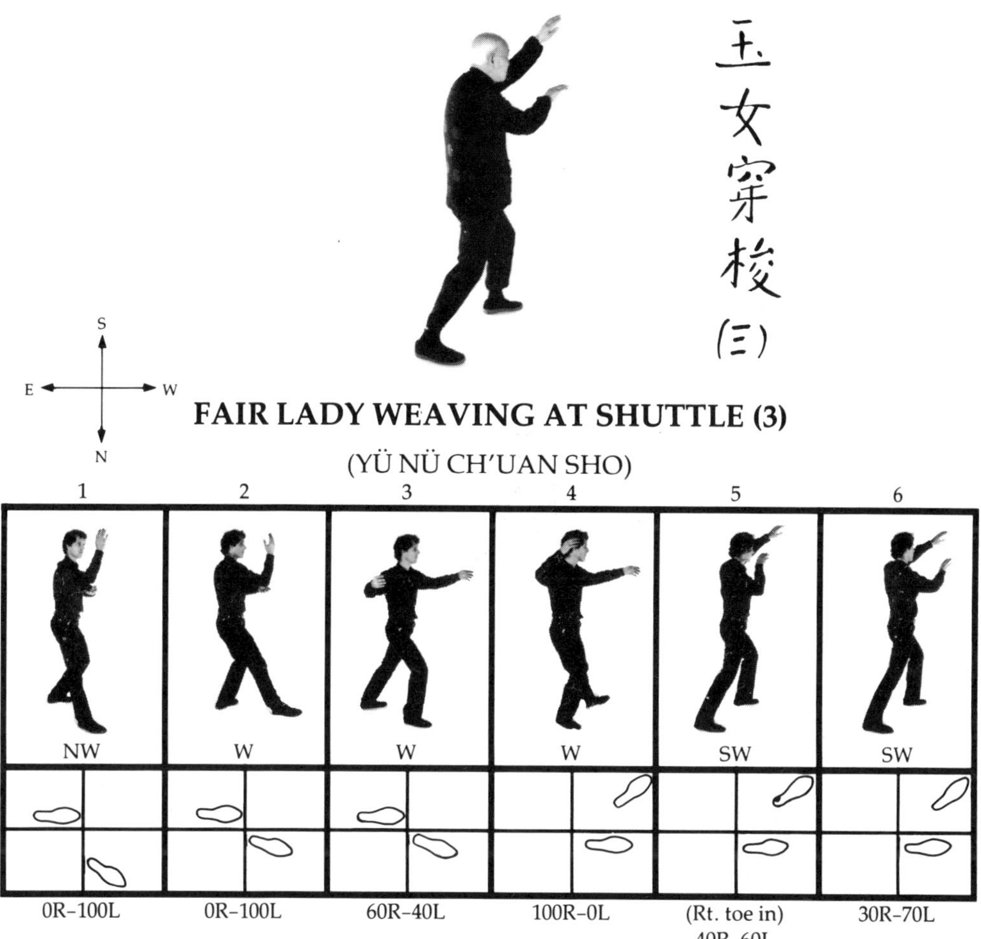

FAIR LADY WEAVING AT SHUTTLE (3)

(YÜ NÜ CH'UAN SHO)

During the Counts of:

1. Shift your weight to the left foot, and bending your right arm, bring your right hand near your right ear with palm facing southwest, and lower your left hand near the right side of your waist under the right elbow with the palm upward.
2. Shift your right foot about three inches to the left, setting the heel down first with the toes pointing northwest.
3. Shift your weight to the right foot. At the same time begin to circle your right hand counterclockwise, downward and backward, and gradually raise your left hand upward and to the left with the palm facing you.
4. Step with your left foot forward and leftward (southwest) with the heel touching first. Continue to circle your right hand upward and forward and stop it beside your right ear with the palm forward.
5. Begin to shift your weight to your left foot and gradually turn your body to the left (to face southwest). At the same time continue to raise your left hand

upward and over your forehead, turning the palm outward with the elbow slightly bent. Turn your right foot slightly inward. The right hand continues to circle, palm outward, to the front of the body.

6. Shift 70% of your weight to the left foot and push forward with your right hand together with the energy of your whole body as one unit. Now you are facing southwest.

POSTURE 91

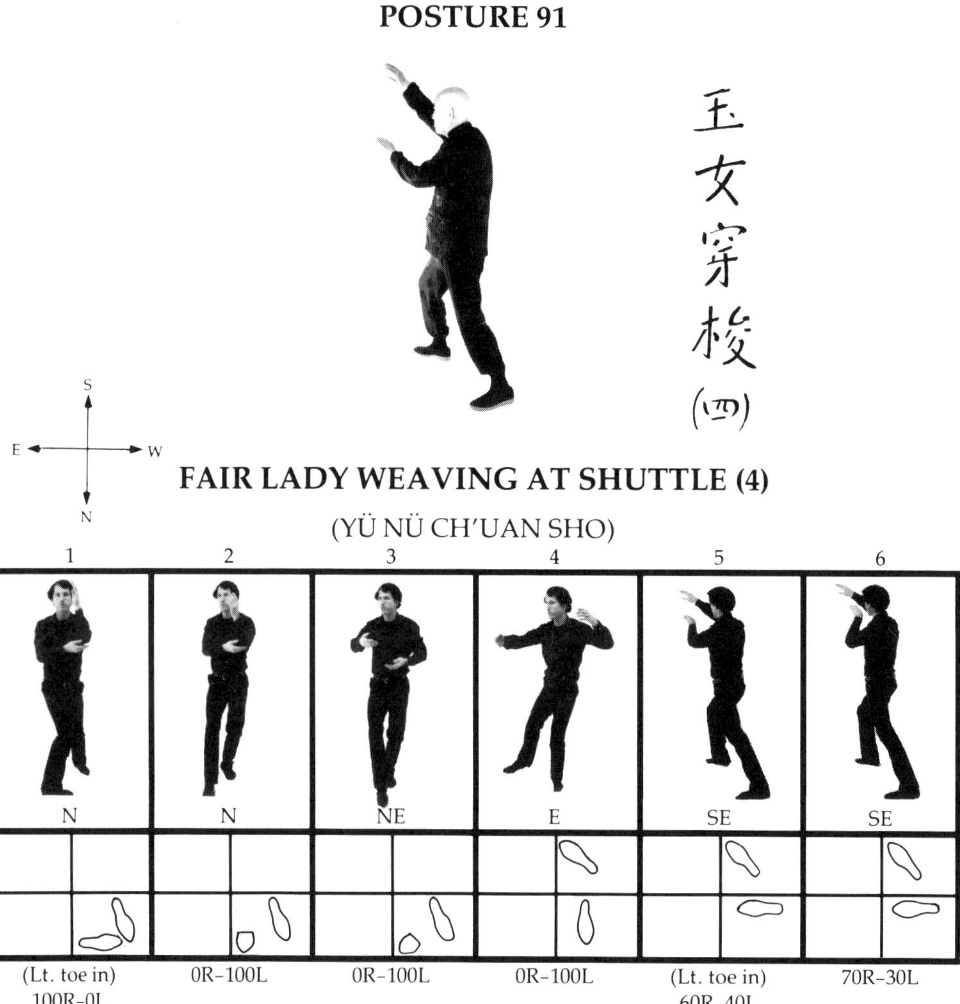

FAIR LADY WEAVING AT SHUTTLE (4)

(YÜ NÜ CH'UAN SHO)

During the Counts of:

1. Shift your weight to the right foot, and gradually turn your body to the right (to face north) while pivoting on the left heel turning the left foot inward so that it points north. At the same time bend your left arm and bring your left hand near your left ear, with the palm facing northeast. Lower your right hand near your left waist to a position under your left elbow, with the palm upward.

2. Shift your weight to the left foot so that your right foot is raised to its toes pointing north.
3. Begin to raise your right hand rightward and upward with the palm facing you and circle your left hand clockwise, downward and backward. At the same time gradually turn your body to the right (to northeast).
4. Step with your right foot forward and rightward, with the heel touching first so that the toes finish pointing southeast. At the same time continue to circle your left hand upward and forward and stop it near your left ear with the palm forward and continue to raise your right hand to head level.
5. Gradually shift your weight to the right foot and continue to turn your body to the right (to face southeast). At the same time raise your right hand over your forehead and turn your palm outward with the elbow slightly bent. Turn your left foot slightly inward. The left hand circles forward to the front of the body, palm outward.
6. Shift 70% of your weight to the right foot and push forward with your left hand together with the energy of your whole body as one unit. Now you are facing southeast.

POSTURE 92

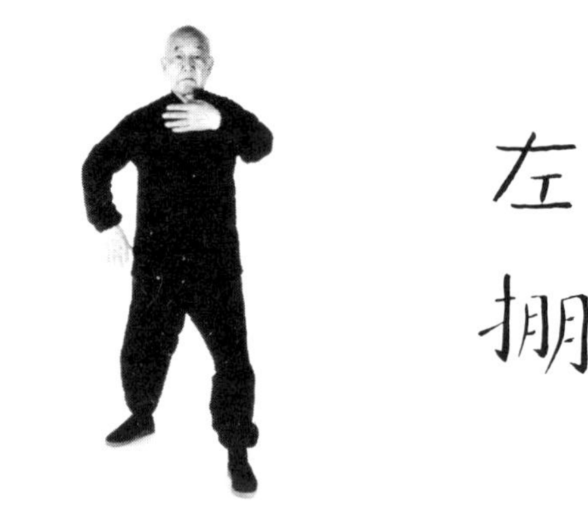

WARD OFF, LEFT

(TSO P'ENG)

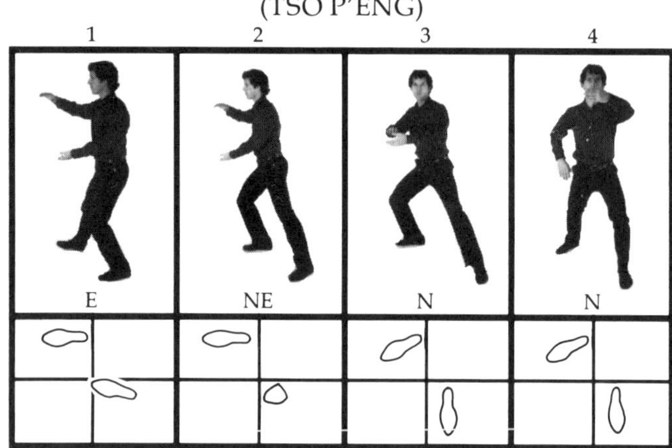

This posture is the same as posture #82.

POSTURE 93

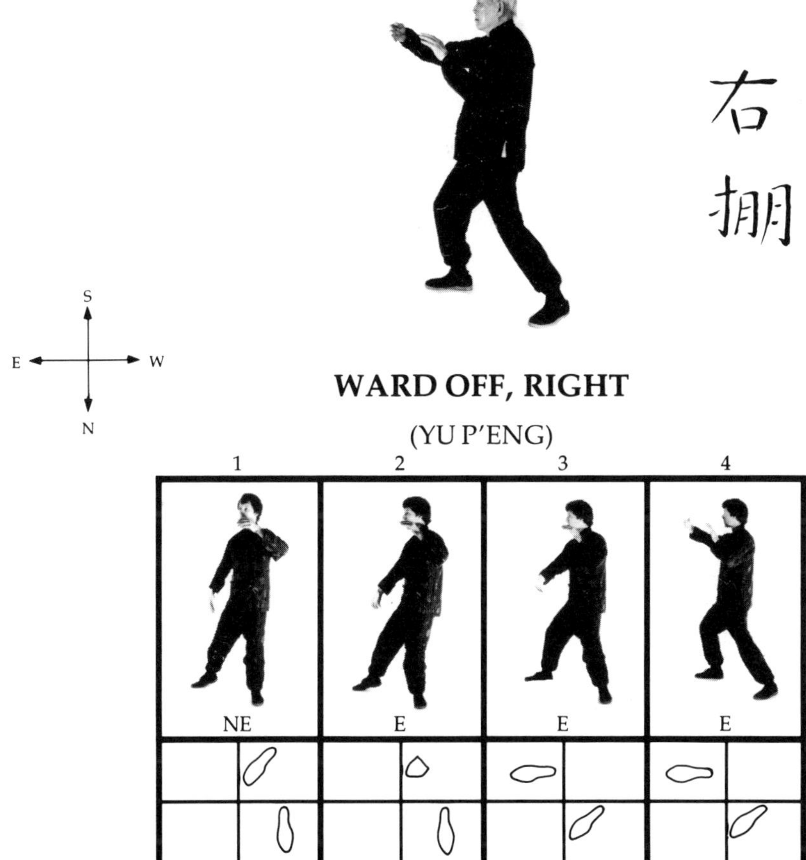

WARD OFF, RIGHT

(YU P'ENG)

This posture is the same as posture #4.

POSTURE 94

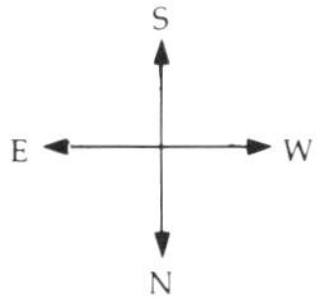

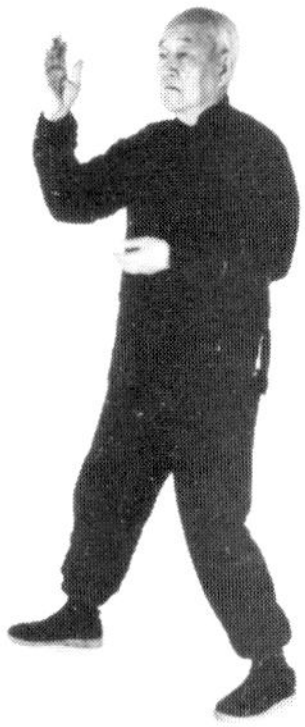

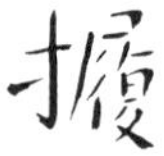

ROLL BACK

(LÜ)

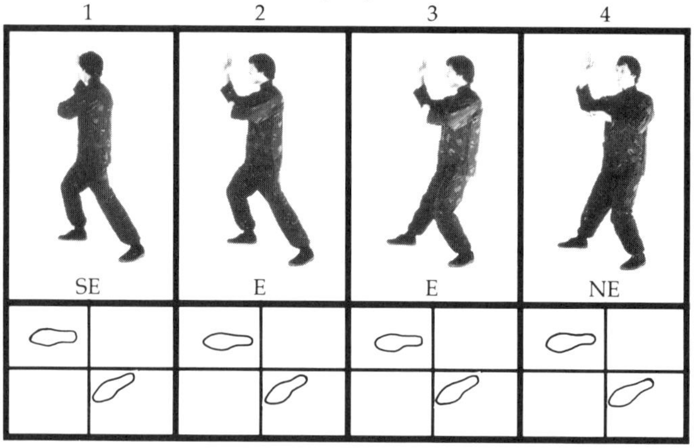

This posture is the same as posture #5.

POSTURE 95

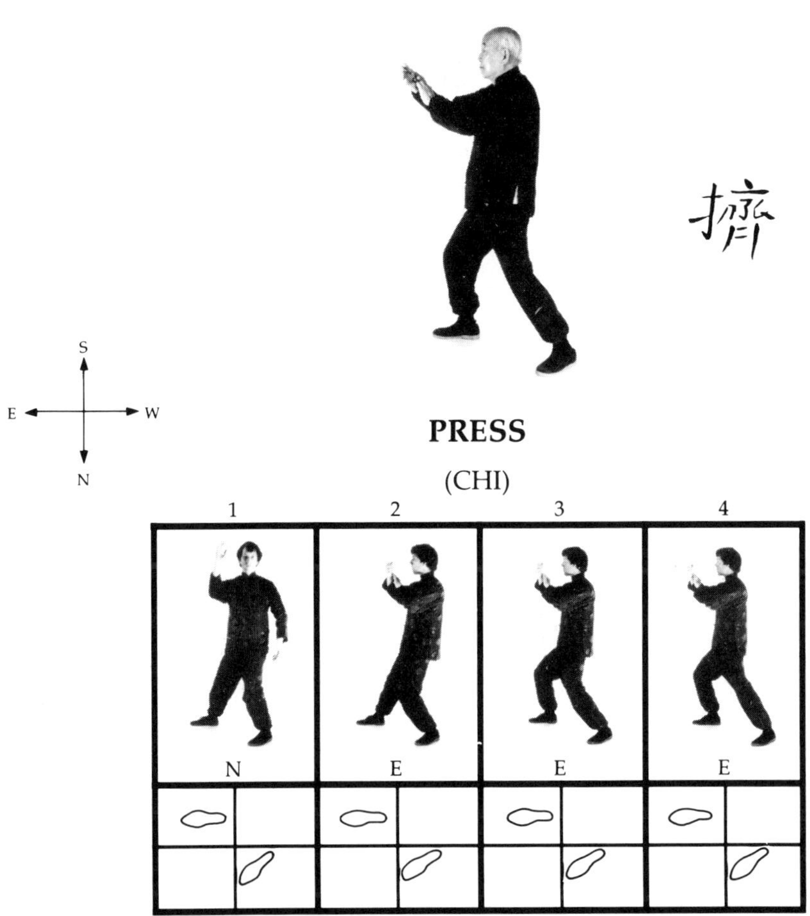

This posture is the same as posture #6.

POSTURE 96

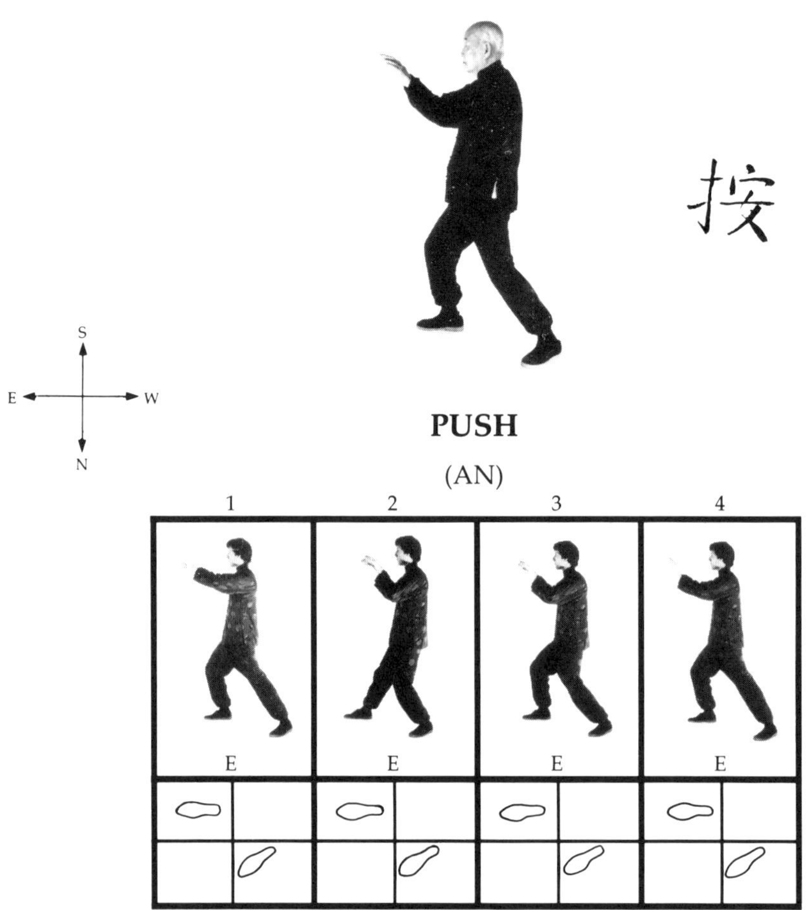

PUSH

(AN)

This posture is the same as posture #7.

POSTURE 97

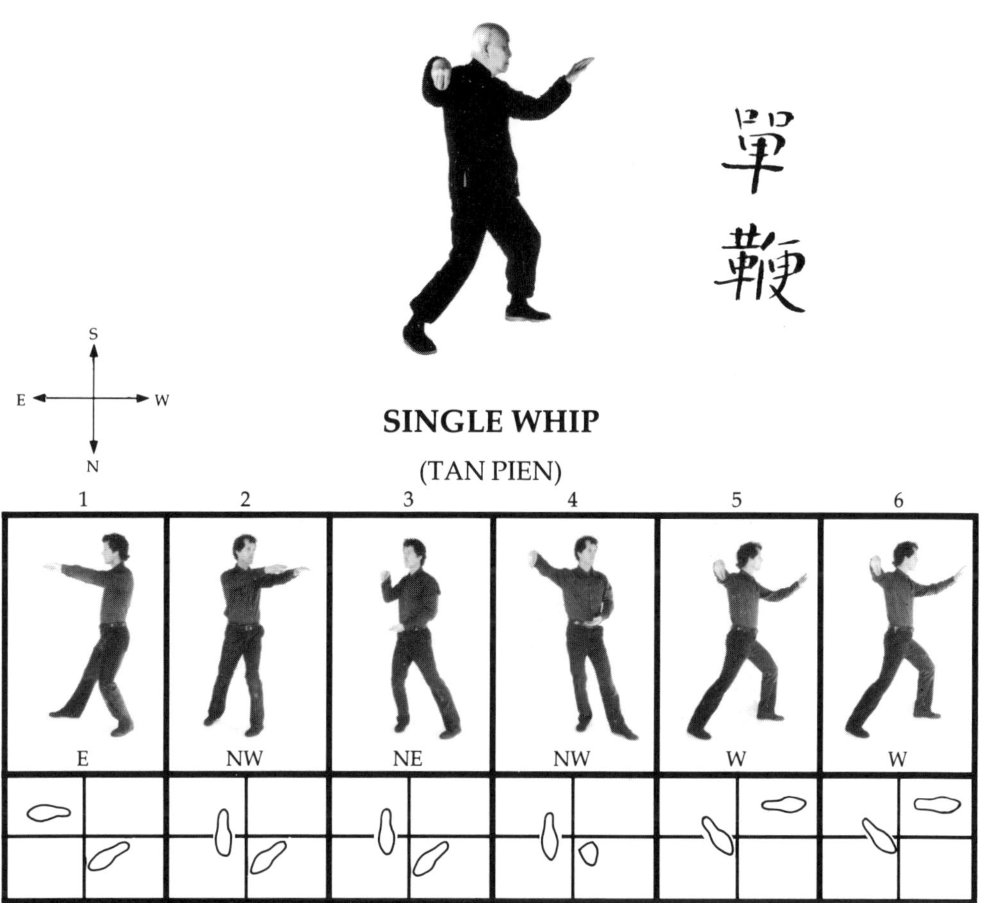

SINGLE WHIP

(TAN PIEN)

This posture is the same as posture #8.

POSTURE 98

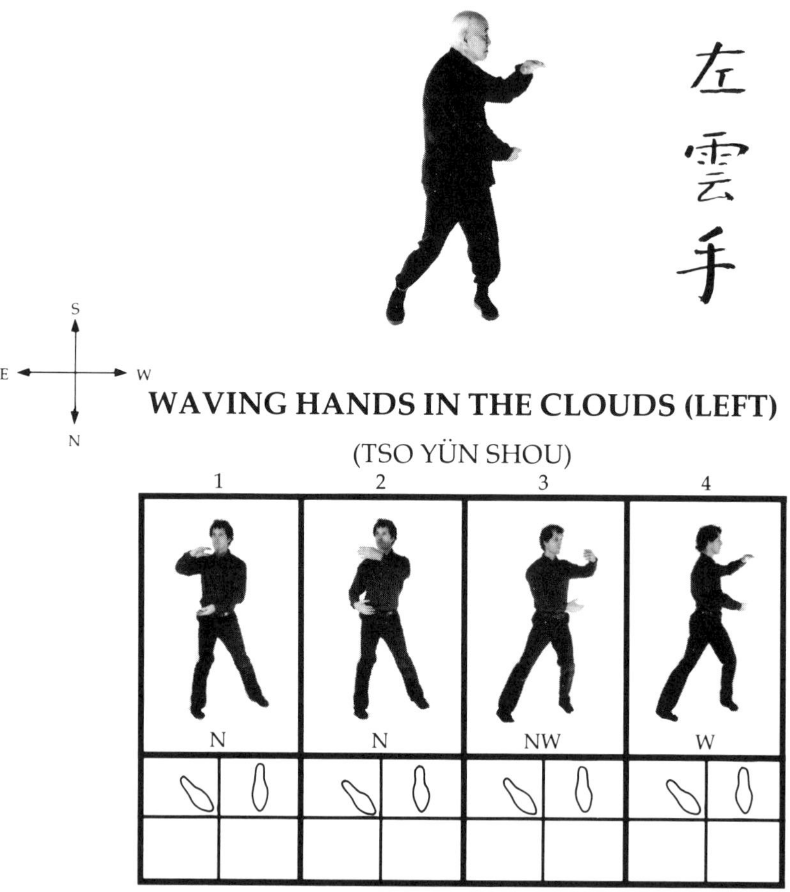

WAVING HANDS IN THE CLOUDS (LEFT)

(TSO YÜN SHOU)

This posture is the same as posture #48.

POSTURE 99

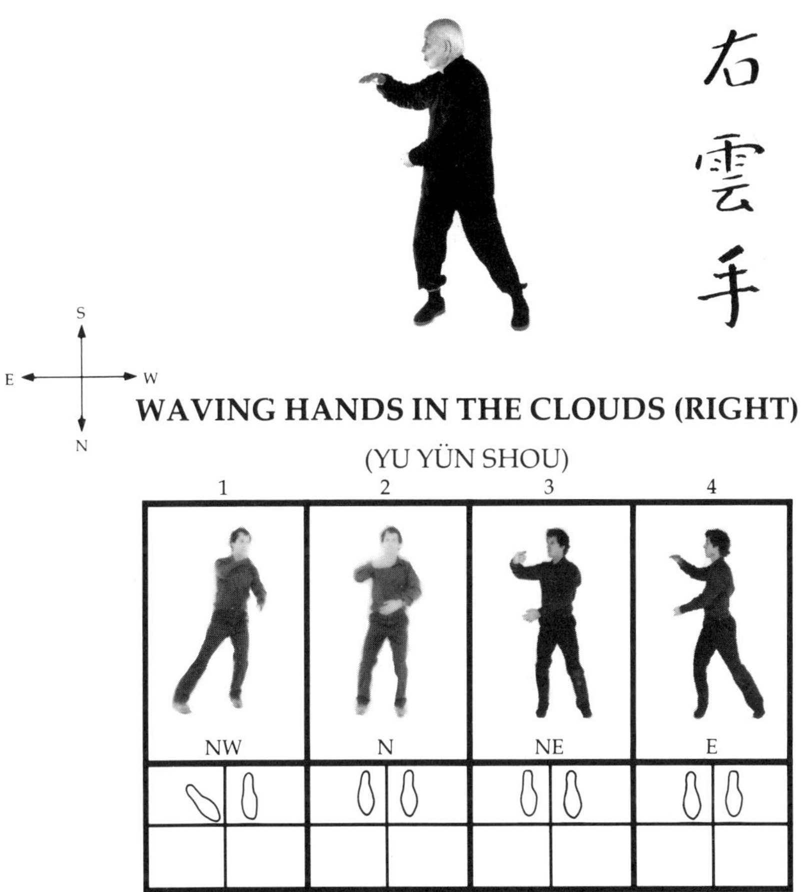

WAVING HANDS IN THE CLOUDS (RIGHT)

(YU YÜN SHOU)

This posture is the same as posture #49.

POSTURE 100

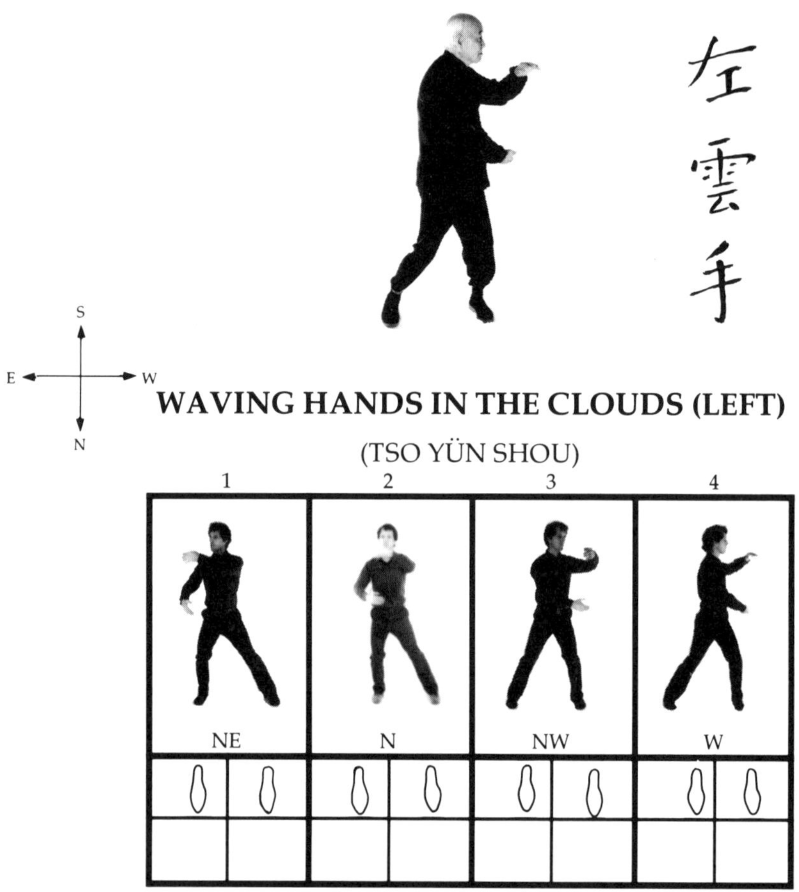

WAVING HANDS IN THE CLOUDS (LEFT)

(TSO YÜN SHOU)

This posture is the same as posture #50.

POSTURE 101

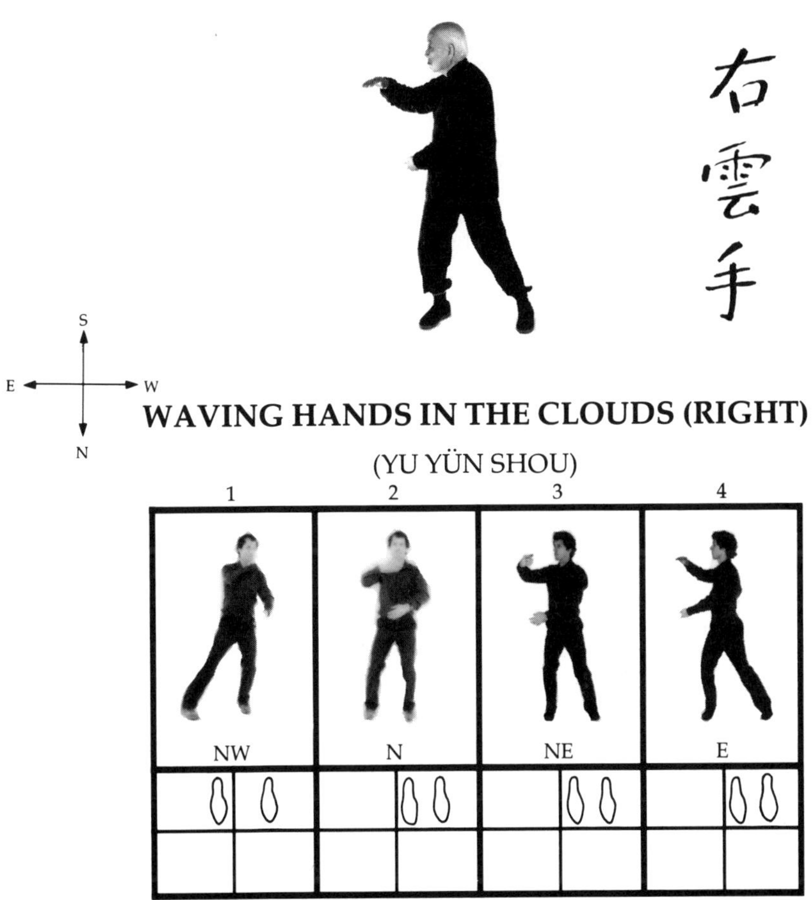

WAVING HANDS IN THE CLOUDS (RIGHT)

(YU YÜN SHOU)

This posture is the same as posture #49.

POSTURE 102

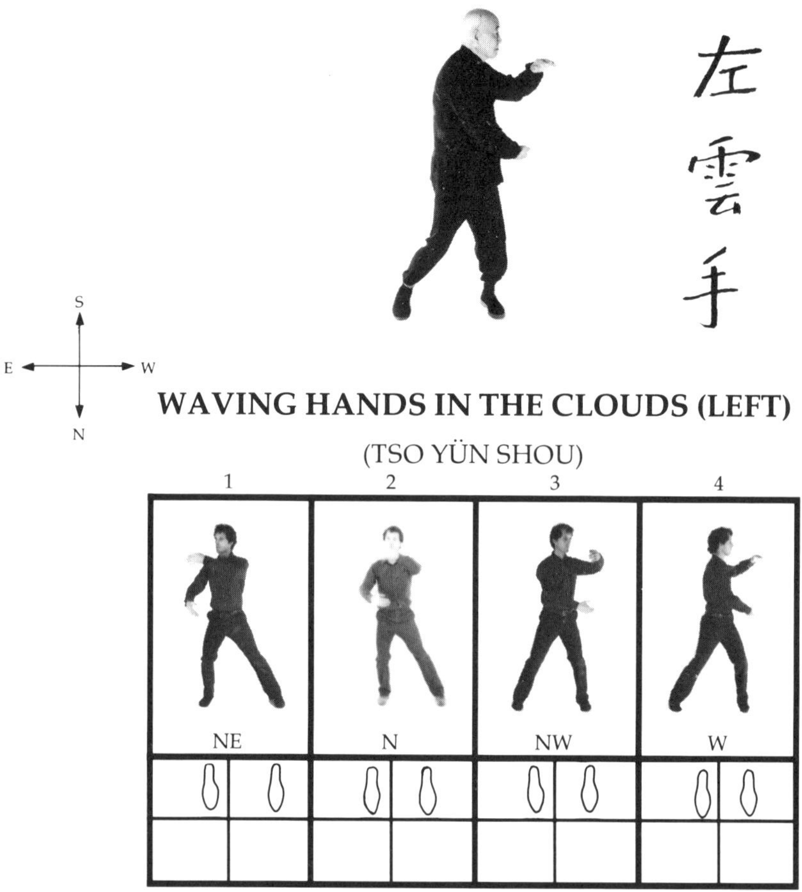

WAVING HANDS IN THE CLOUDS (LEFT)

(TSO YÜN SHOU)

This posture is the same as posture #50.

POSTURE 103

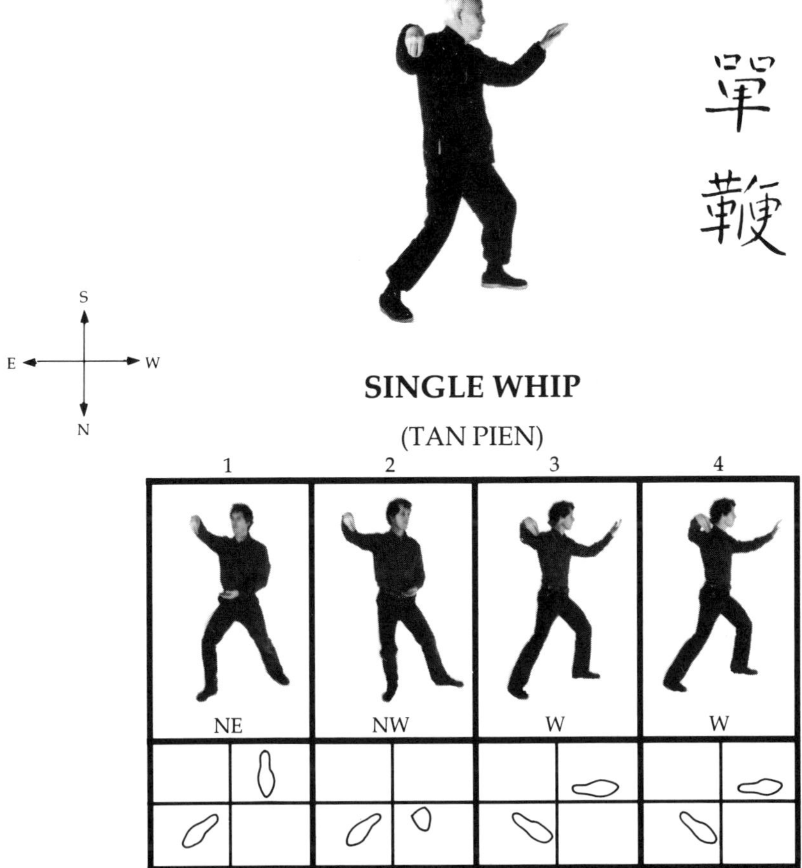

SINGLE WHIP

(TAN PIEN)

This posture is the same as posture #53.

POSTURE 104

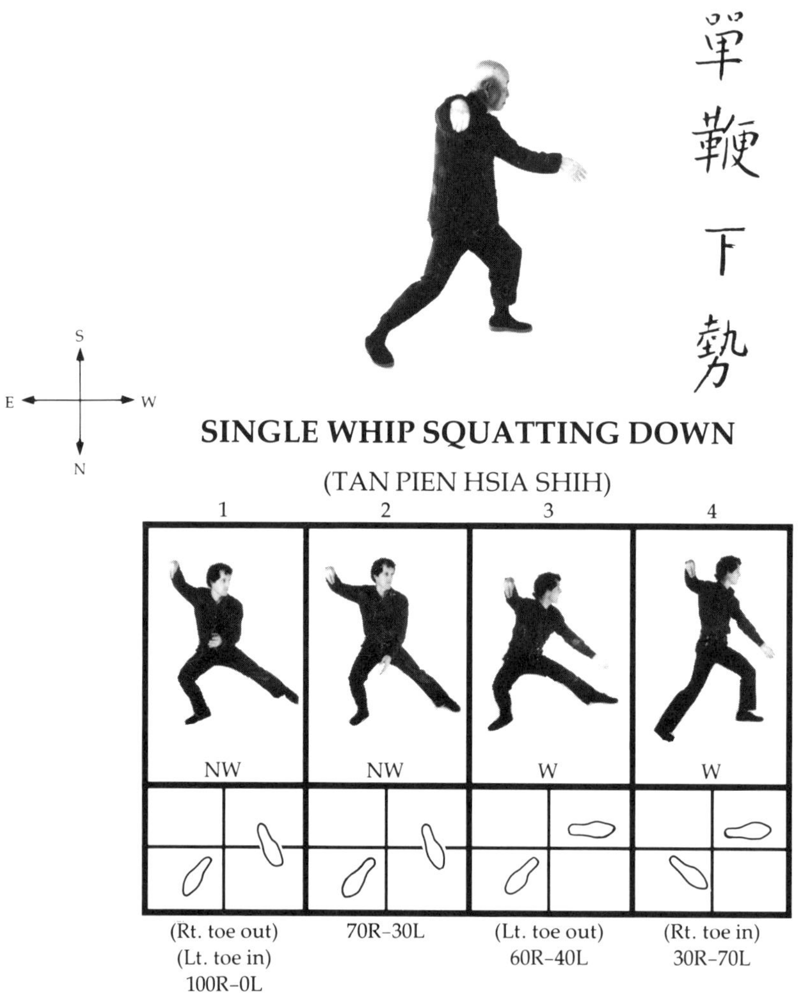

SINGLE WHIP SQUATTING DOWN

(TAN PIEN HSIA SHIH)

During the Counts of:

1. Turn your right foot on its heel 90 degrees to the right with the toes pointing northeast. Draw back and shift all your weight to your right leg and deeply bend the knee; lower your body so that you almost sit on your right foot. At the same time turn your left foot 45 degrees inward to the right so that the toes point northwest. Draw back your left hand near your right thigh with the palm facing east.
2. Begin to shift your weight to the left leg. The waist begins to turn to the left at this time and the left arm starts to drop during its arcing movement.
3. Turn your left foot, pivoting on the heel, 45 degrees to the left so that the toes point west. At the same time lower your left hand so that it traces an arc down along the left knee and forward with the palm facing north.
4. Slowly shift 70% of your weight to the left foot by bending the left knee and straightening the right knee. Turn your right foot 90 degrees inward, pointing it northwest. Your right hand is still kept hooked behind you (toward the northeast) to maintain balance and your left hand continues forward with the palm facing north. You are now facing west.

POSTURE 105

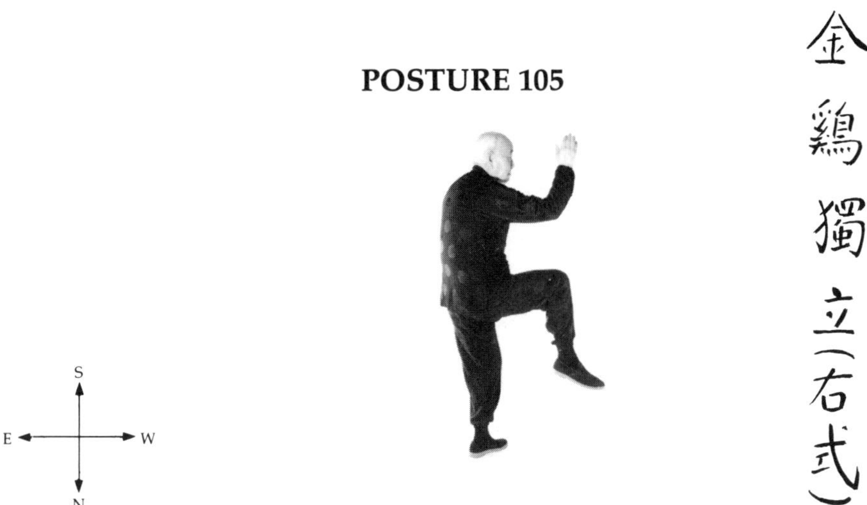

GOLDEN ROOSTER STANDING ON ONE LEG (RIGHT)

(CHIN CHI TU LI, YU SHIH)

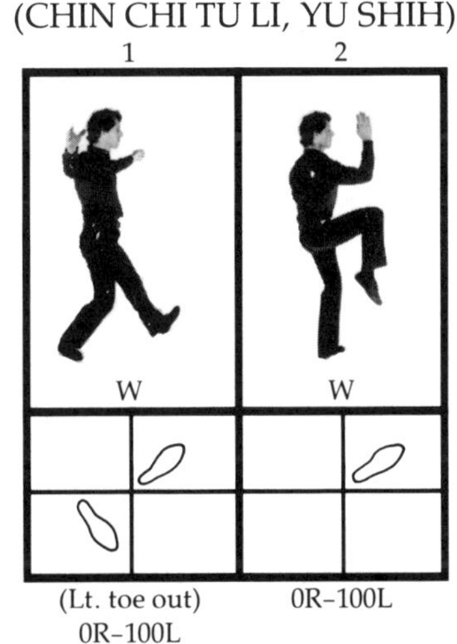

(Lt. toe out) 0R-100L | 0R-100L

During the Counts of:

1. Shift the weight to the right leg and turn the left foot out (SW). Shift your weight entirely to your left leg and keeping it slightly bent, lower your left hand beside your left thigh with the palm backward. At the same time open your right "hook hand" and lower it beside your right thigh with the palm inward. (Note: This photograph does not show the completion of the beat. It shows only the weight shift onto the back leg and toe out of left foot.)
2. Raise your right hand forward and up to head level with the elbow bent, fingers pointing up and the palm facing south. At the same time lift your right foot forward and upward with the knee bent and toes pointing down so that your right elbow is above your right knee, forming a perpendicular line from knee to hand. You are still facing west.

POSTURE 106

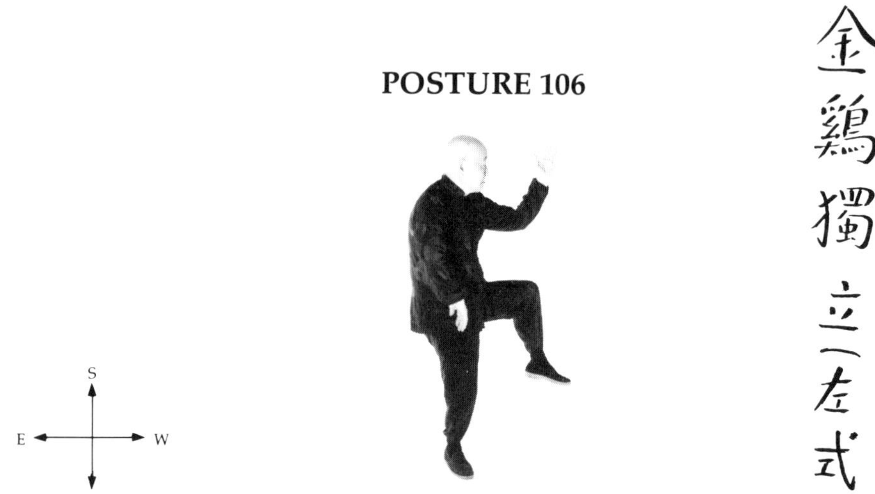

GOLDEN ROOSTER STANDING ON ONE LEG (LEFT)

(CHIN CHI TU LI, TSO SHIH)

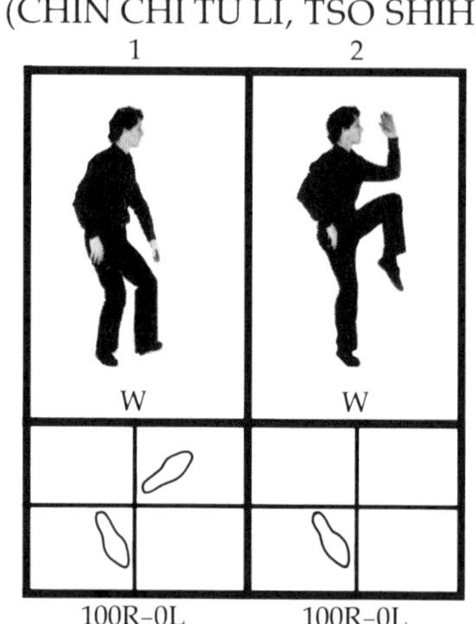

During the Counts of:

1. Take a half step backward with your right foot, setting it down turned slightly outward, and shift the weight to it with the knee slightly bent. At the same time lower your right hand and put it beside your right thigh with the palm backward.
2. Raise your left hand forward up to head level with the elbow bent, fingers pointing up and palm facing north. At the same time lift up your left foot with the toes pointing down and knee bent, so that your left elbow is above your left knee forming a perpendicular line. You are still facing west.

POSTURE 107

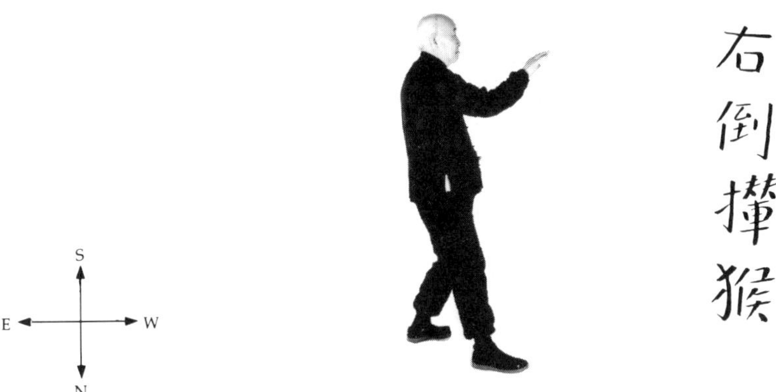

STEP BACK TO DRIVE THE MONKEY AWAY (RIGHT)

(TAO NIEN HOU, YU SHIH)

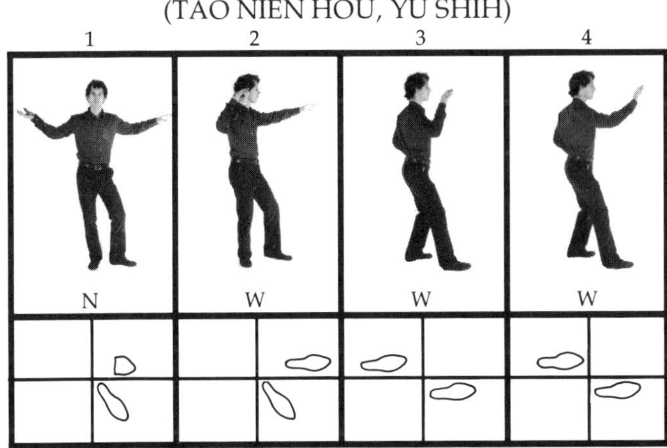

During the Counts of:

1. Lower your left foot in front of your right foot with only the toes touching the ground. Turn your body to the right (to face north). At the same time extend your left arm forward at shoulder height with the palm down and circle your right hand counterclockwise, backward and upward to shoulder height with the palm upward.

Beats 2, 3 and 4 are the same as the respective beats of posture #29.

POSTURE 108

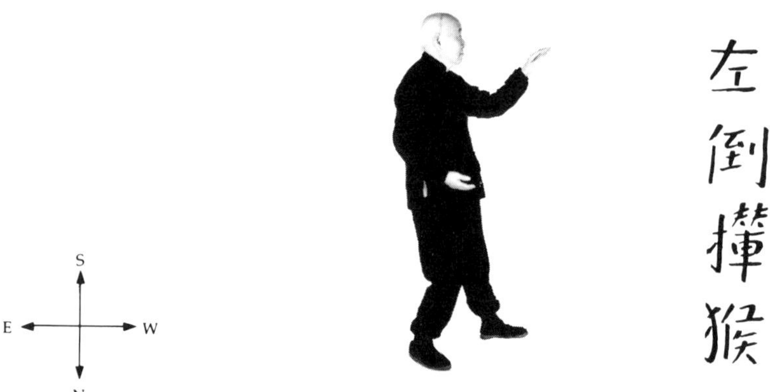

STEP BACK TO DRIVE THE MONKEY AWAY (LEFT)

(TAO NIEN HOU, TSO SHIH)

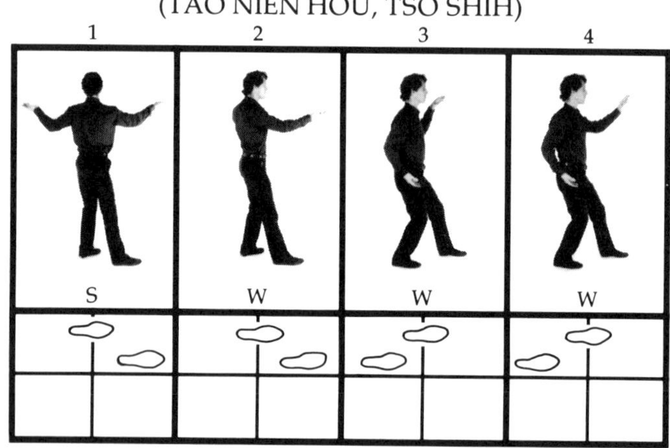

This posture is the same as posture #30.

POSTURE 109

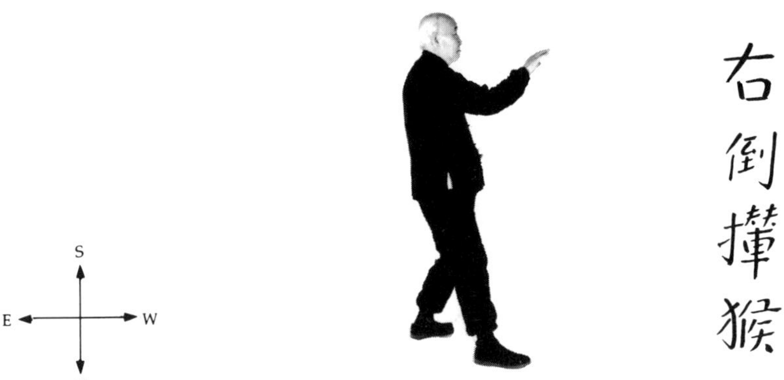

STEP BACK TO DRIVE THE MONKEY AWAY (RIGHT)

(TAO NIEN HOU, YU SHIH)

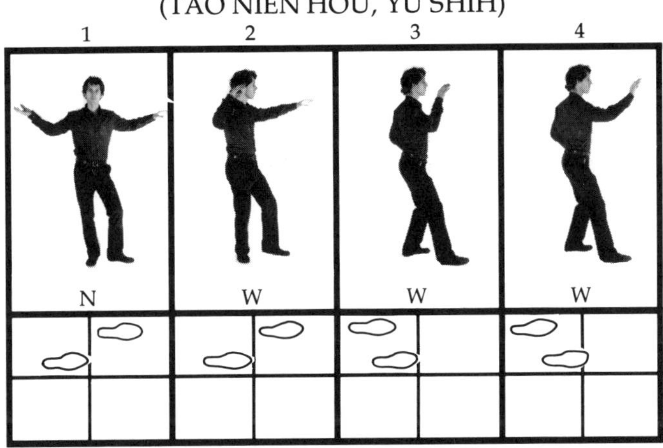

This posture is the same as posture #31.

POSTURE 110

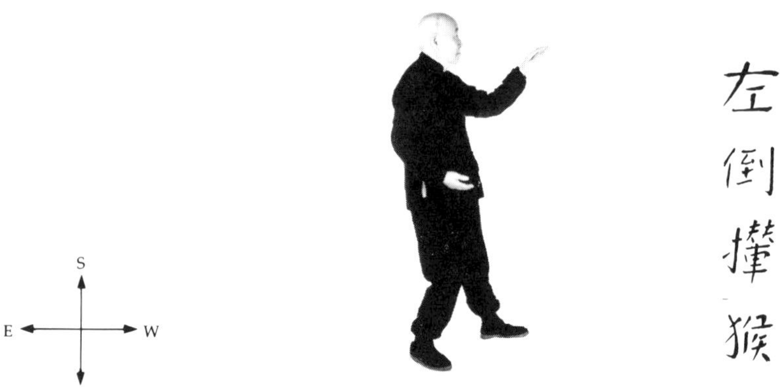

STEP BACK TO DRIVE THE MONKEY AWAY (LEFT)

(TAO NIEN HOU, TSO SHIH)

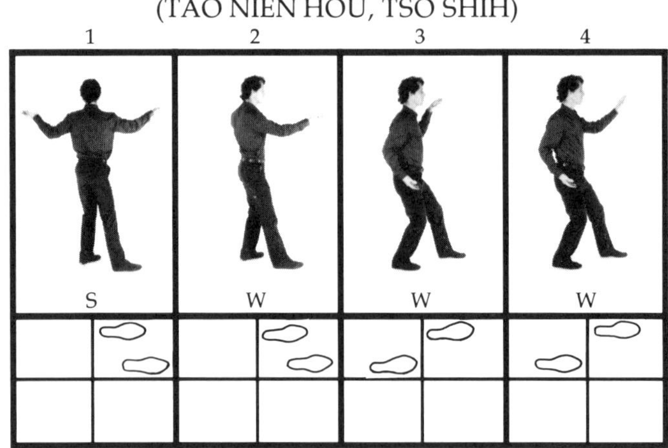

This posture is the same as posture #32.

POSTURE 111

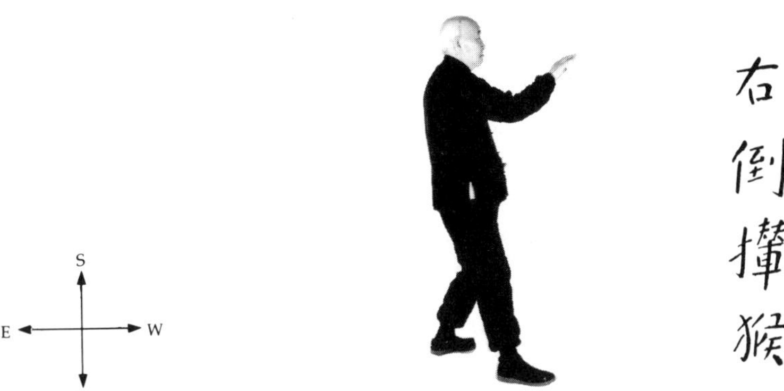

右倒攆猴

STEP BACK TO DRIVE THE MONKEY AWAY (RIGHT)

(TAO NIEN HOU, YU SHIH)

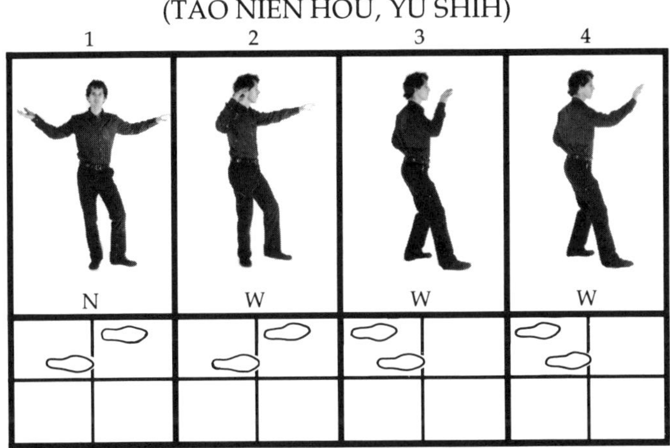

This posture is the same as posture #33.

POSTURE 112

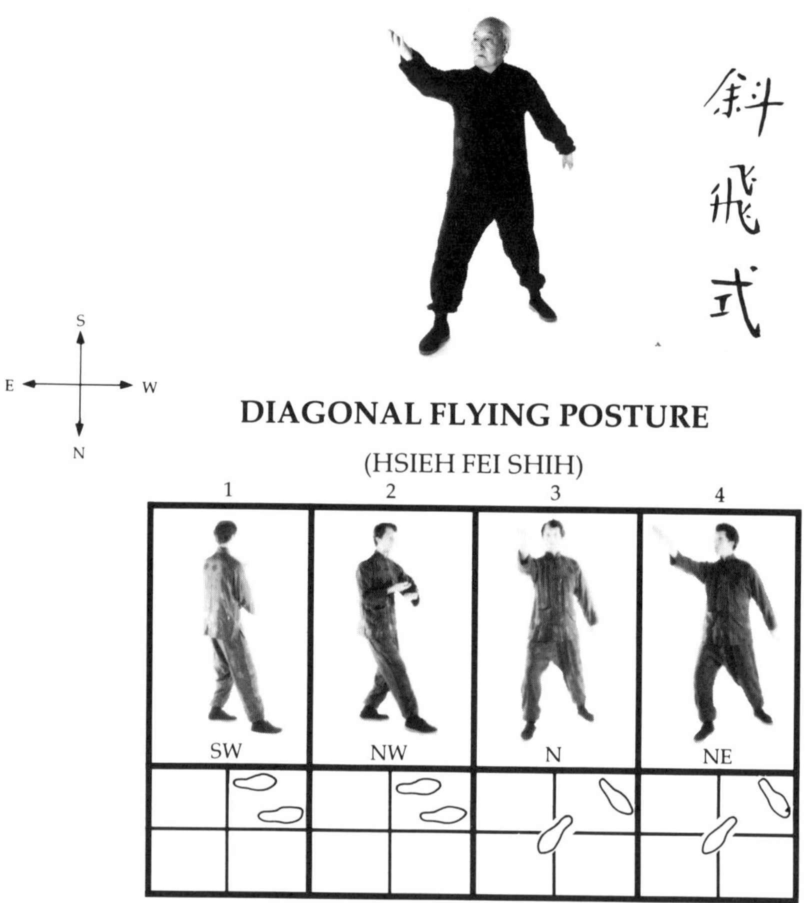

DIAGONAL FLYING POSTURE

(HSIEH FEI SHIH)

This posture is the same as posture #34.

POSTURE 113

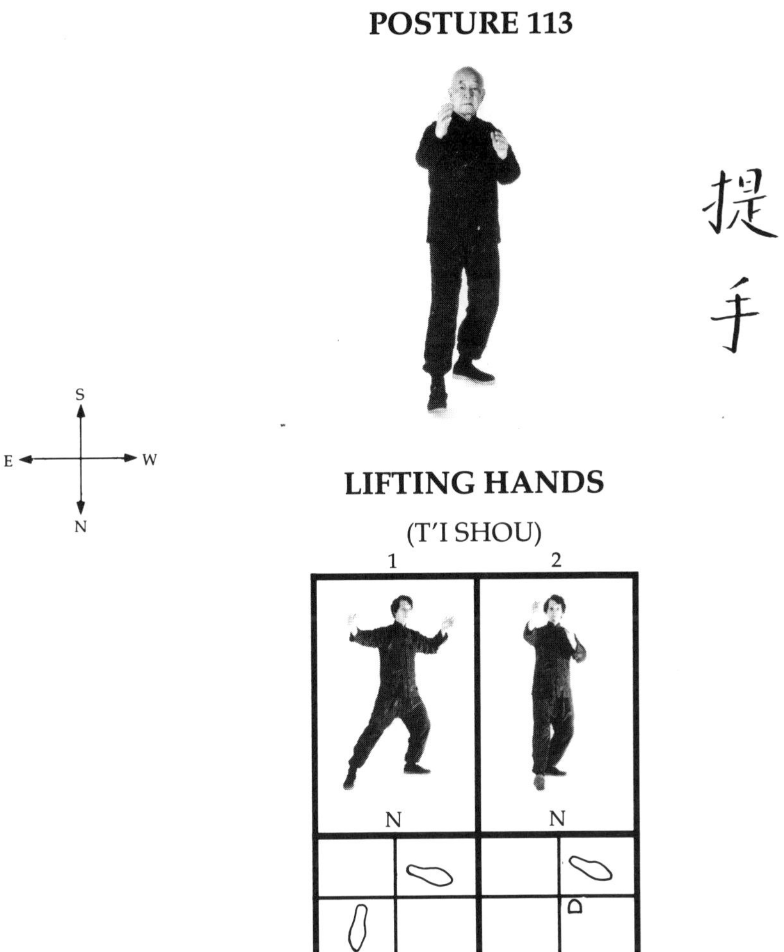

LIFTING HANDS

(T'I SHOU)

This posture is the same as posture #35.

POSTURE 114

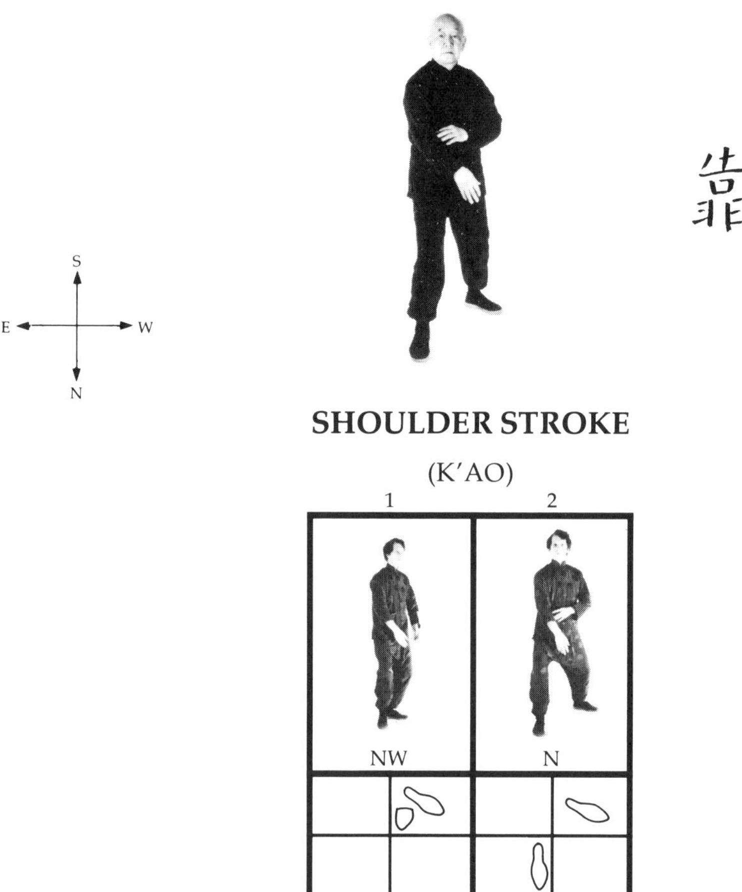

SHOULDER STROKE

(K'AO)

This posture is the same as posture #10.

POSTURE 115

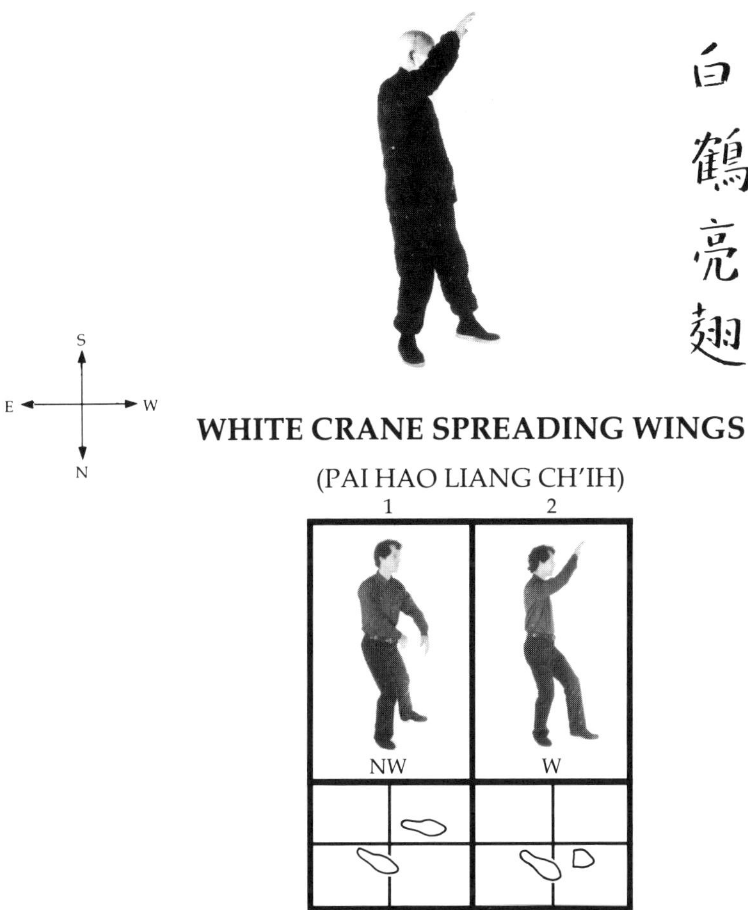

白鶴亮翅

WHITE CRANE SPREADING WINGS

(PAI HAO LIANG CH'IH)

This posture is the same as posture #11.

POSTURE 116

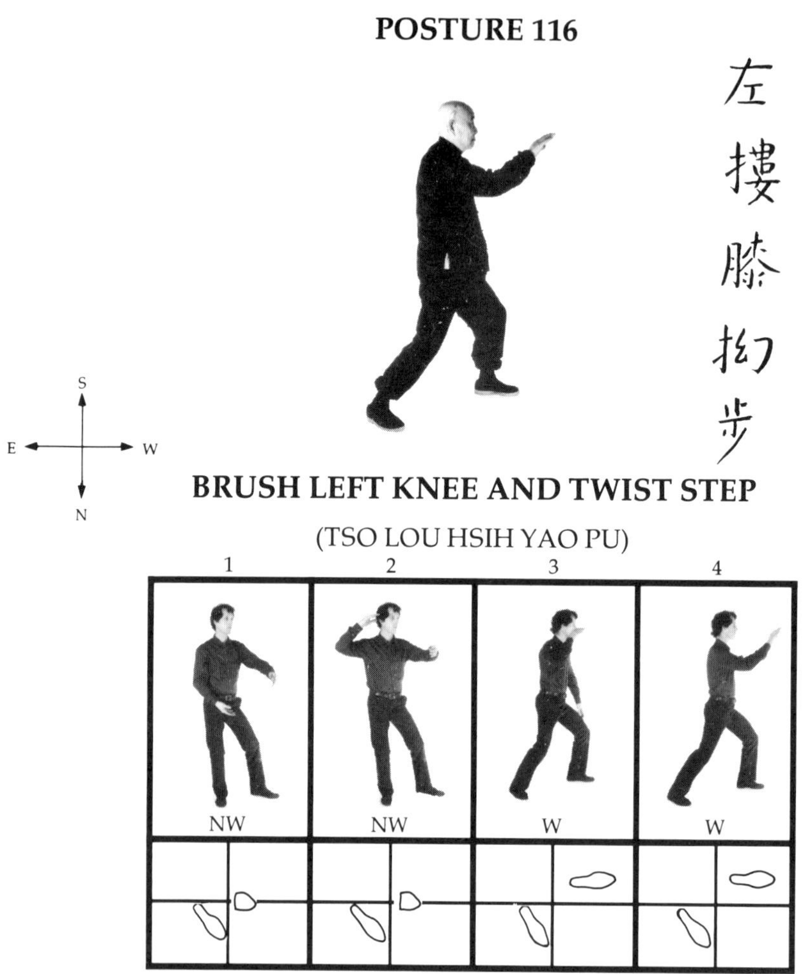

BRUSH LEFT KNEE AND TWIST STEP

(TSO LOU HSIH YAO PU)

This posture is the same as posture #12.

POSTURE 117

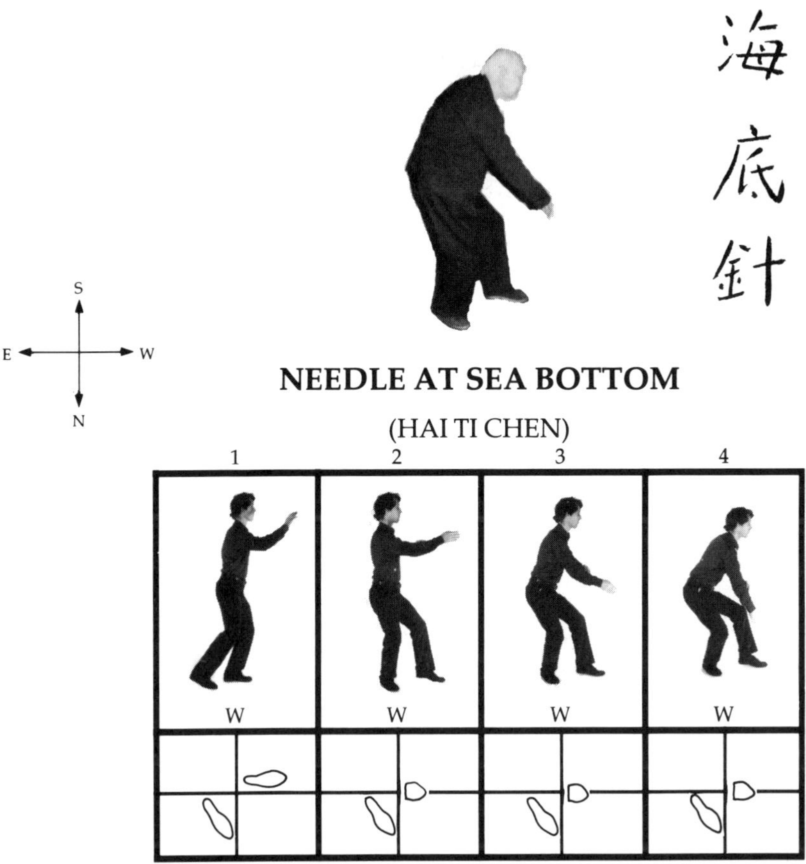

NEEDLE AT SEA BOTTOM

(HAI TI CHEN)

This posture is the same as posture #39.

POSTURE 118

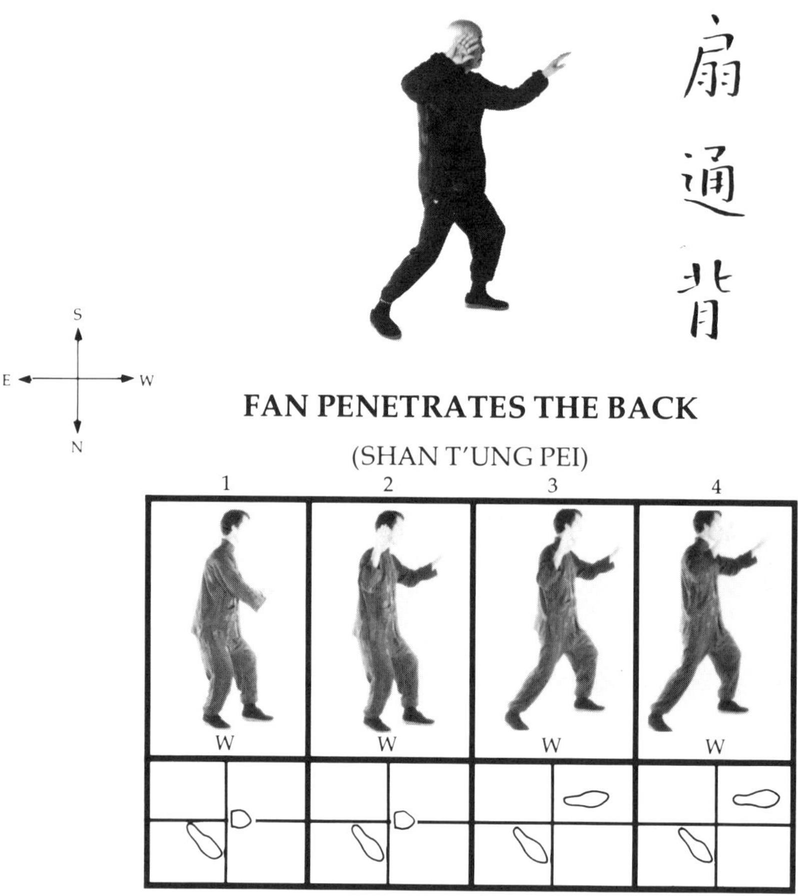

FAN PENETRATES THE BACK

(SHAN T'UNG PEI)

This posture is the same as posture #40.

POSTURE 119

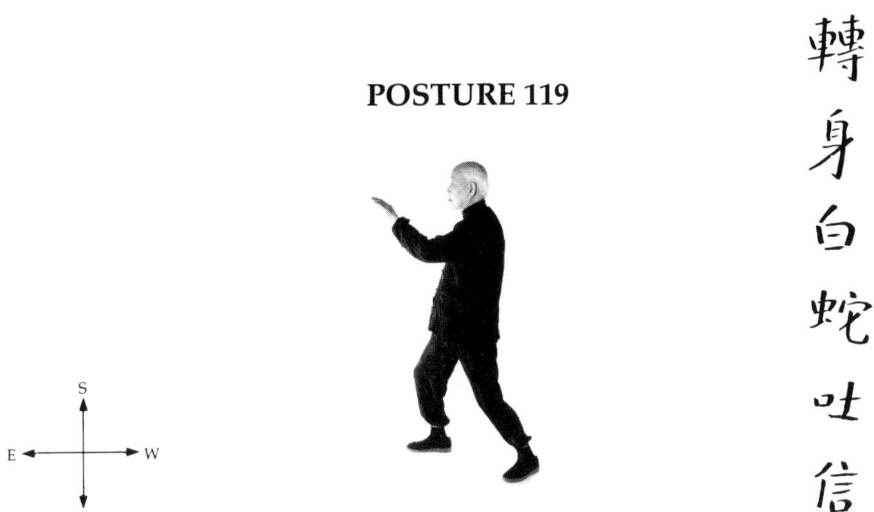

TURN AROUND AND WHITE SNAKE PUTS OUT TONGUE

(CHUAN SHEN PAI SHE T'U HSIN)

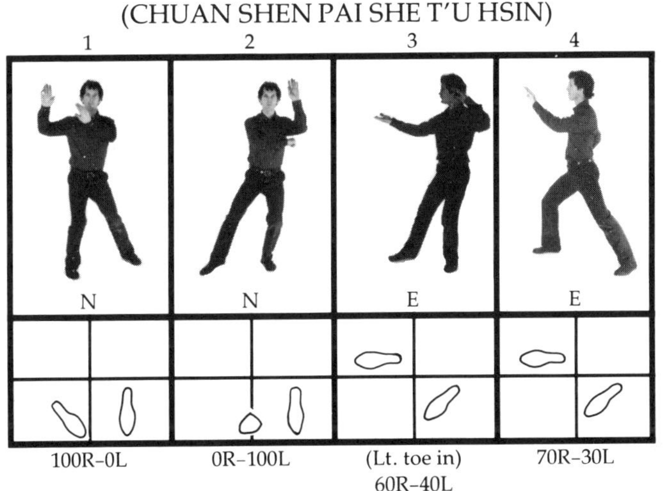

During the Counts of:

1. Circle your hands rightward and turn your body to the right (north). Shift your weight to the right foot. Turn your left foot inward to face north.
2. Continue to circle your hands clockwise downward, leftward and upward, until your left hand is near your left temple with the palm outward and elbow bent. Your right hand forms a fist in front of your chest with the knuckles up. At the same time shift your weight to the left foot, and the right foot is brought to its toes.
3. Turn your body to the right (east) and take a half step in the southeast direction with the right foot with the heel touching first. Open your fist and thrust the fingers forward (east) with palm upward and then draw it back beside your hip joint. At the same time gradually shift your weight to your right foot and turn in your left foot slightly. The left hand circles forward to the front of the body. (Note: the picture shown is not at the end of the beat but part way through to show the extension of the right hand.)

4. Shift 70% of your weight to your right foot. Push forward with your left palm together with the energy of your whole body. You are now facing west.

POSTURE 120

進步搬攔捶

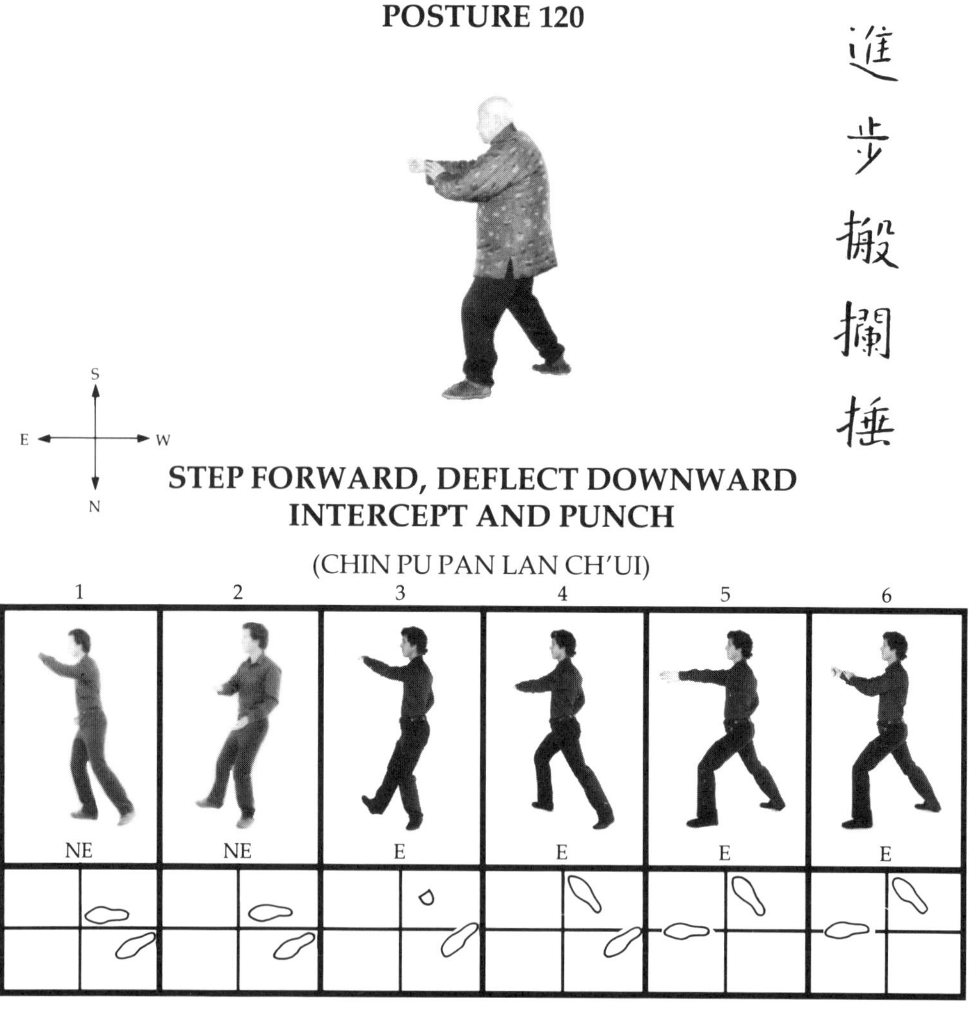

STEP FORWARD, DEFLECT DOWNWARD INTERCEPT AND PUNCH

(CHIN PU PAN LAN CH'UI)

This posture is the same as posture #42.

POSTURE 121

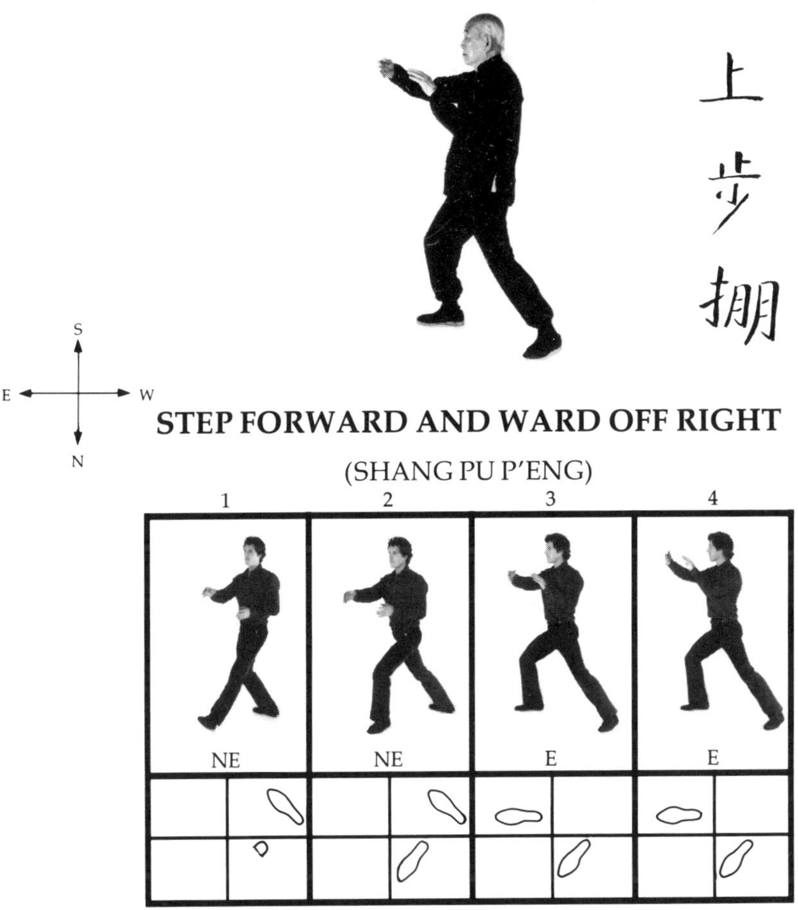

STEP FORWARD AND WARD OFF RIGHT

(SHANG PU P'ENG)

This posture is the same as posture #43.

POSTURE 122

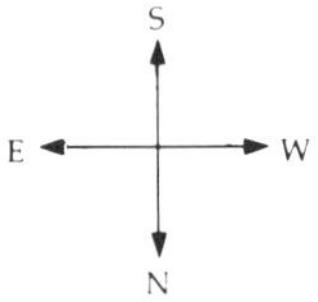

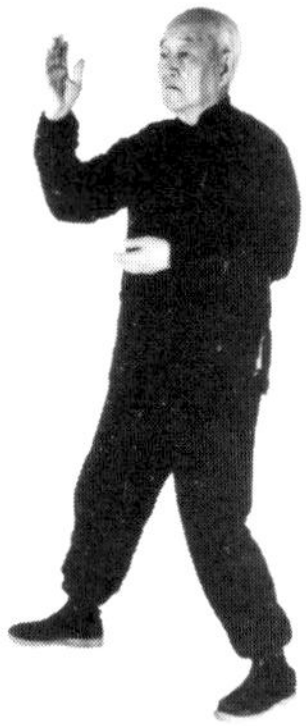

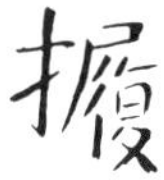

握

S
E W
N

ROLL BACK

(LÜ)

1	2	3	4
SE	E	E	NE

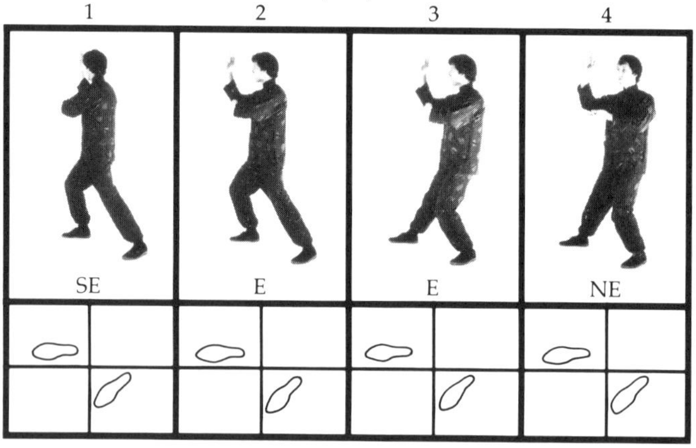

This posture is the same as posture #5.

POSTURE 123

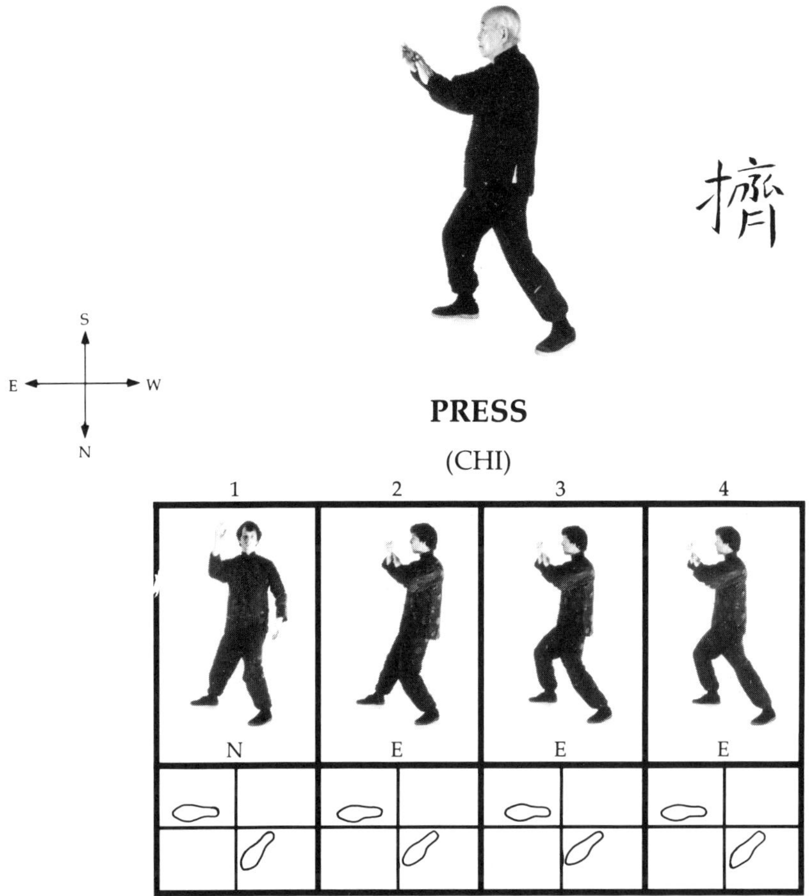

PRESS

(CHI)

This posture is the same as posture #6.

POSTURE 124

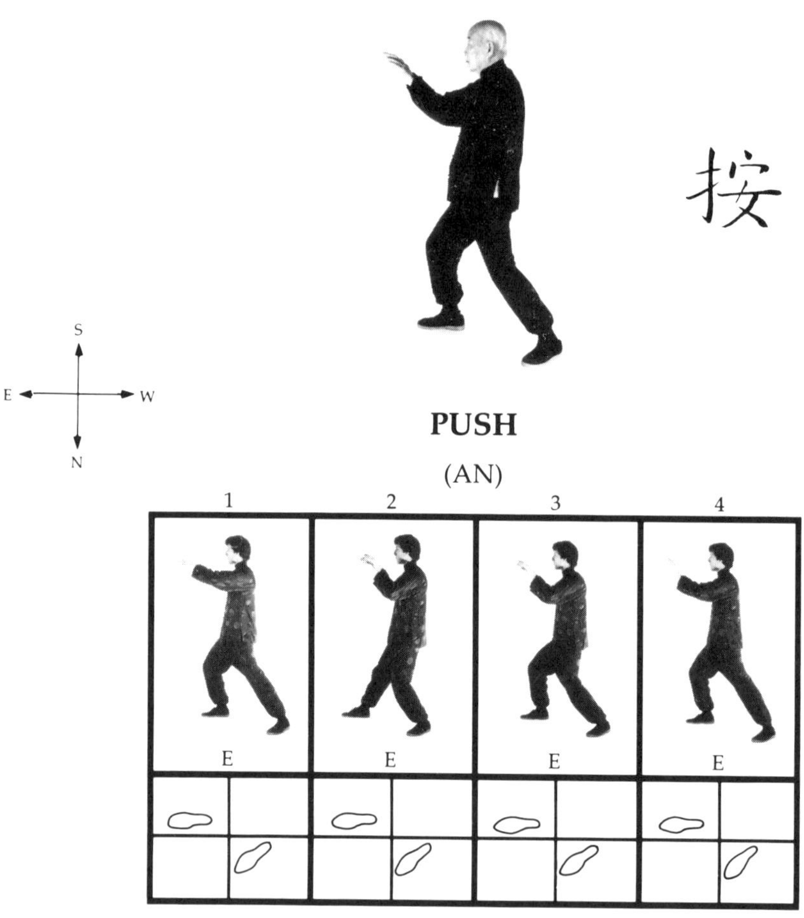

PUSH

(AN)

This posture is the same as posture #7.

POSTURE 125

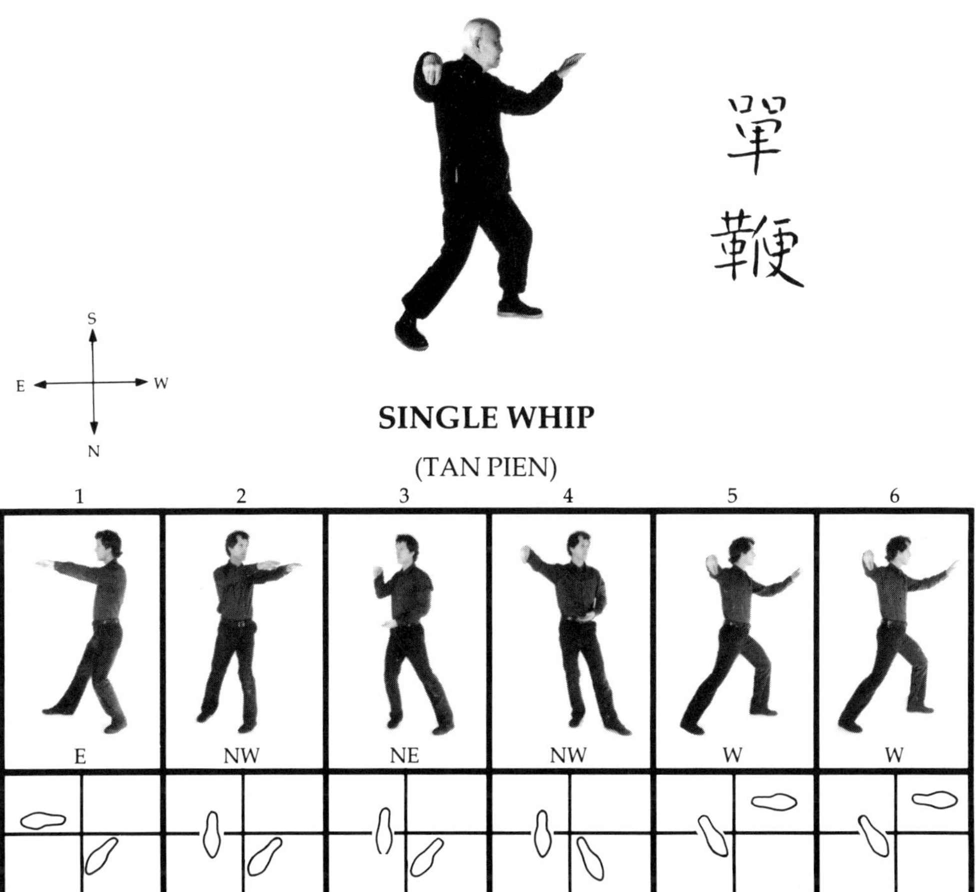

SINGLE WHIP

(TAN PIEN)

This posture is the same as posture #8.

POSTURE 126

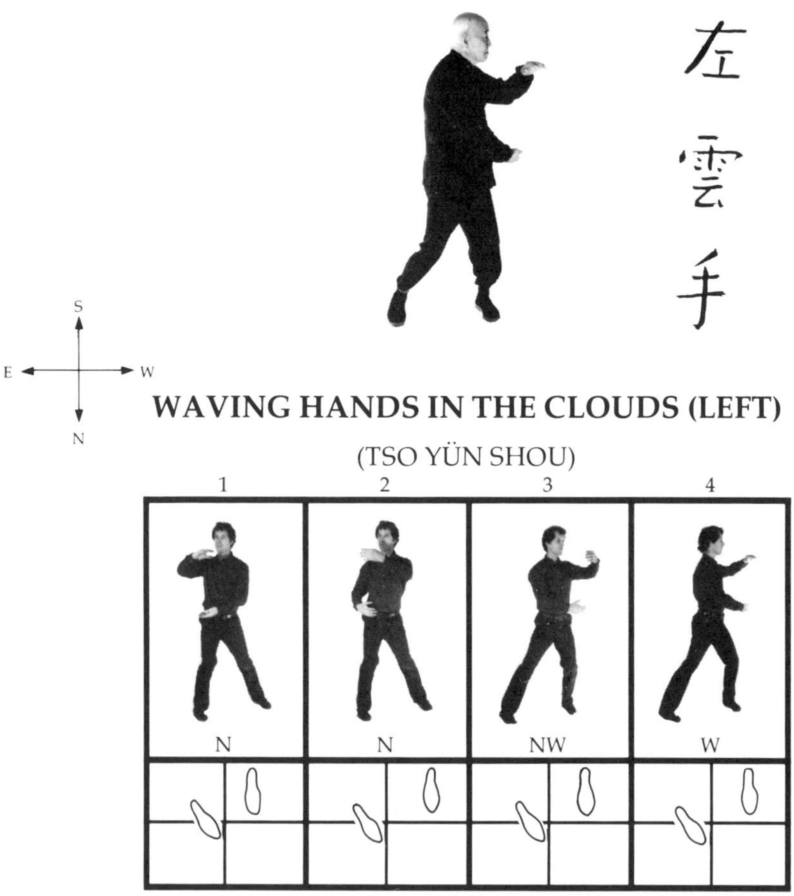

WAVING HANDS IN THE CLOUDS (LEFT)

(TSO YÜN SHOU)

This posture is the same as posture #48.

POSTURE 127

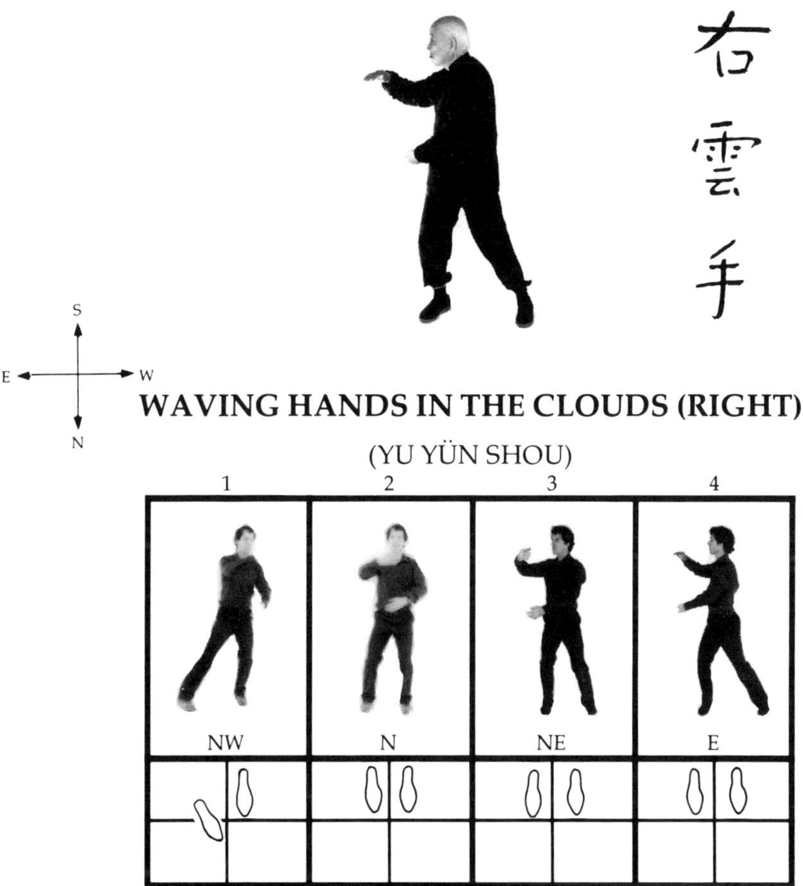

右雲手

WAVING HANDS IN THE CLOUDS (RIGHT)

(YU YÜN SHOU)

This posture is the same as posture #49.

POSTURE 128

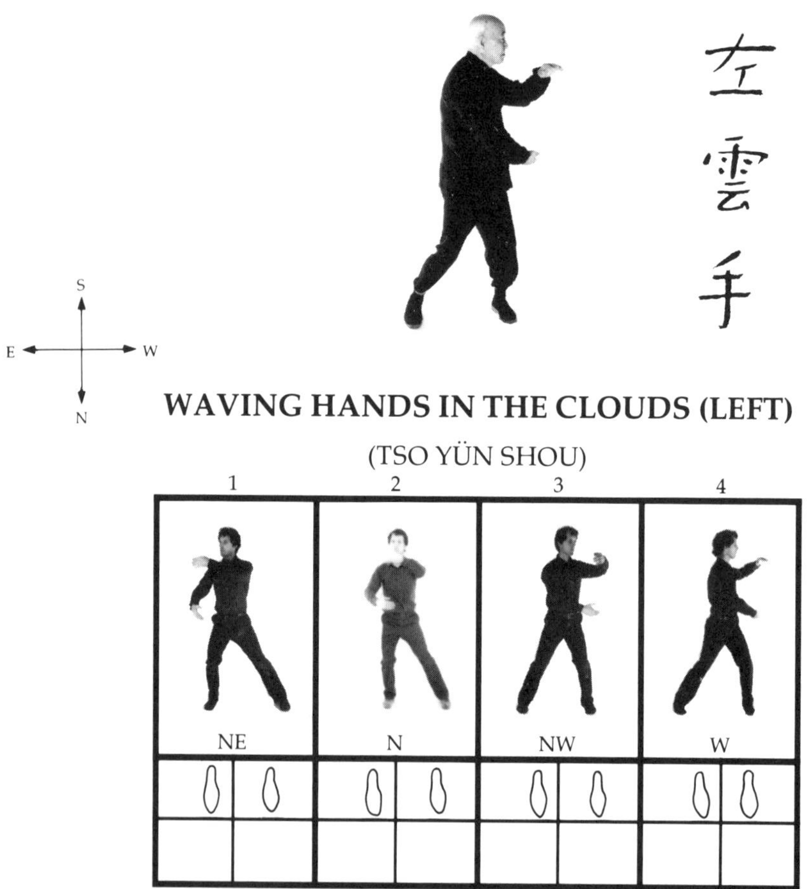

WAVING HANDS IN THE CLOUDS (LEFT)

(TSO YÜN SHOU)

This posture is the same as posture #50.

POSTURE 129

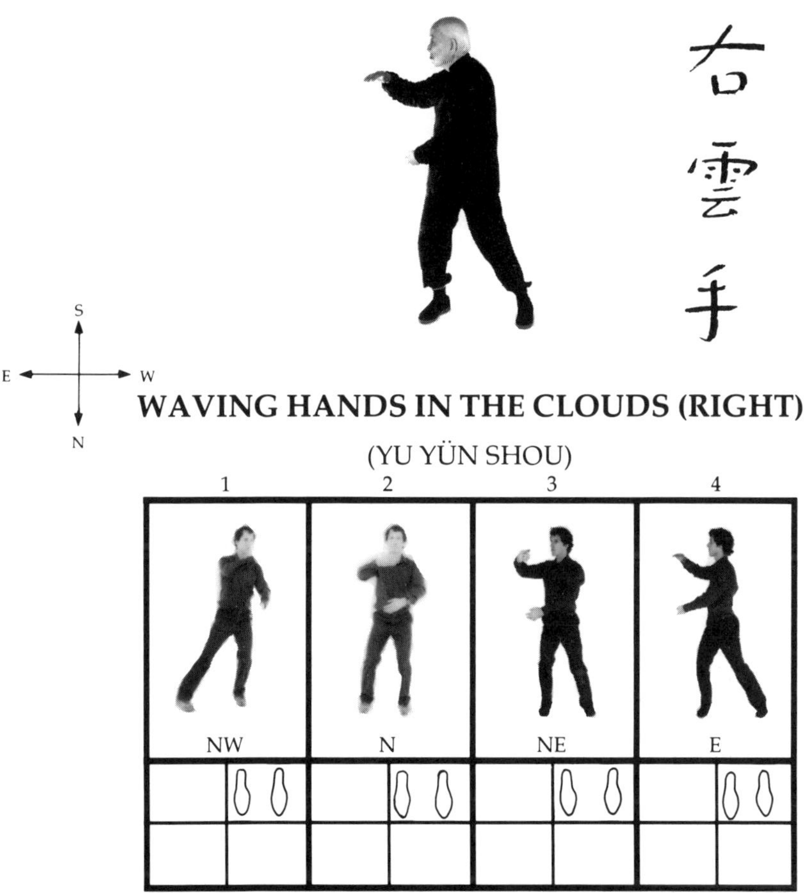

WAVING HANDS IN THE CLOUDS (RIGHT)

(YU YÜN SHOU)

This posture is the same as posture #49.

POSTURE 130

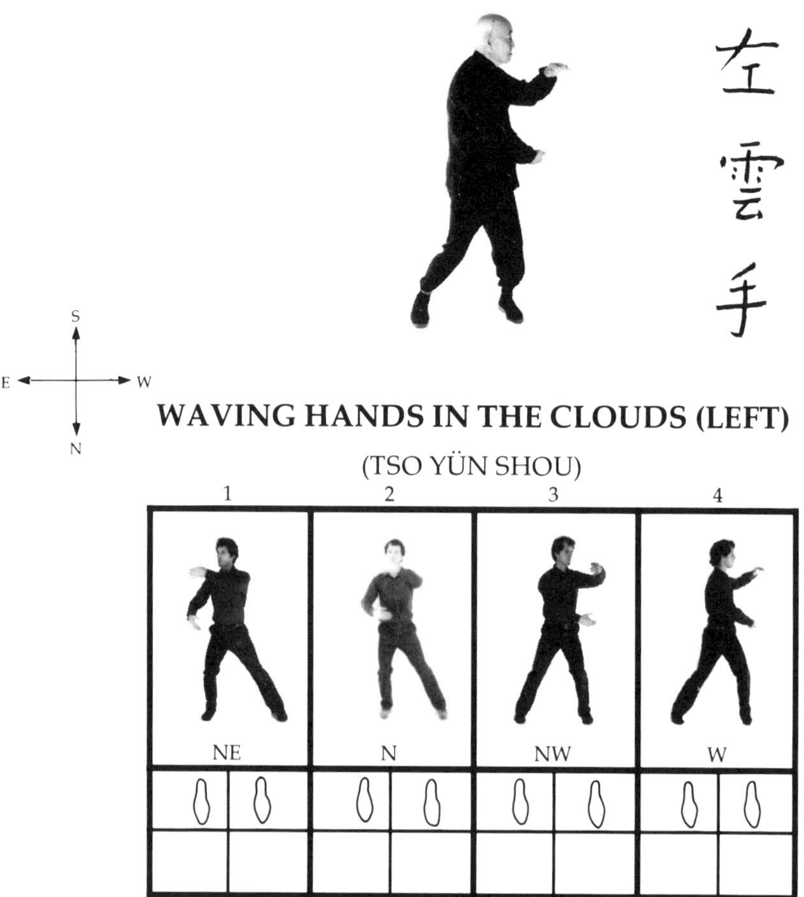

WAVING HANDS IN THE CLOUDS (LEFT)

(TSO YÜN SHOU)

This posture is the same as posture #50.

POSTURE 131

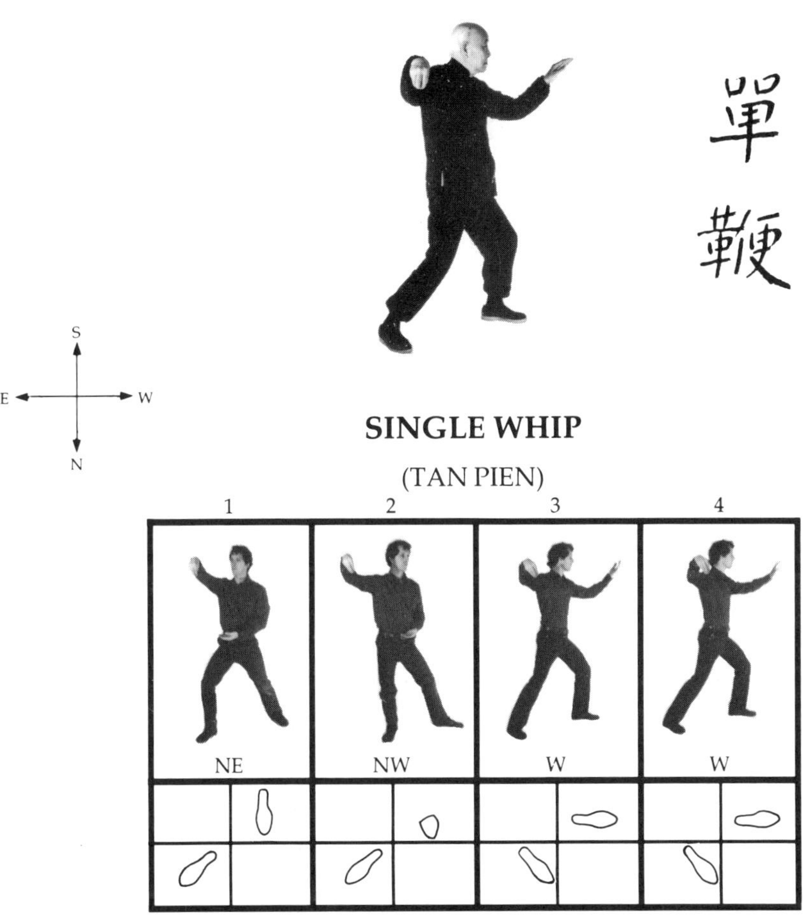

SINGLE WHIP

(TAN PIEN)

This posture is the same as posture #53.

POSTURE 132

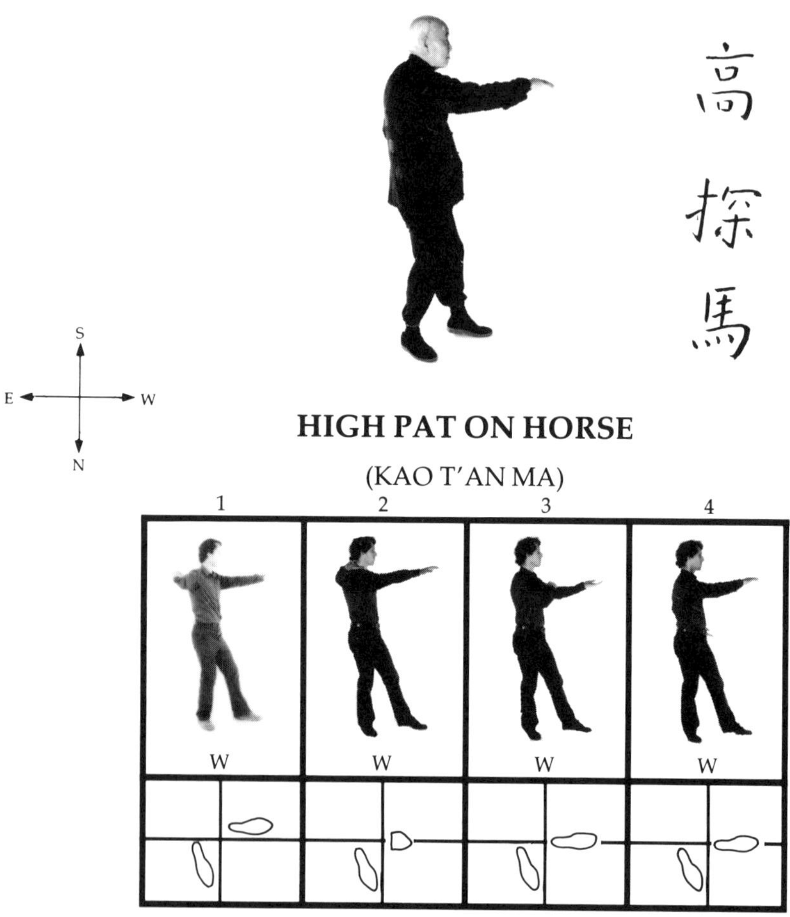

HIGH PAT ON HORSE

(KAO T'AN MA)

This posture is the same as posture #54.

POSTURE 133

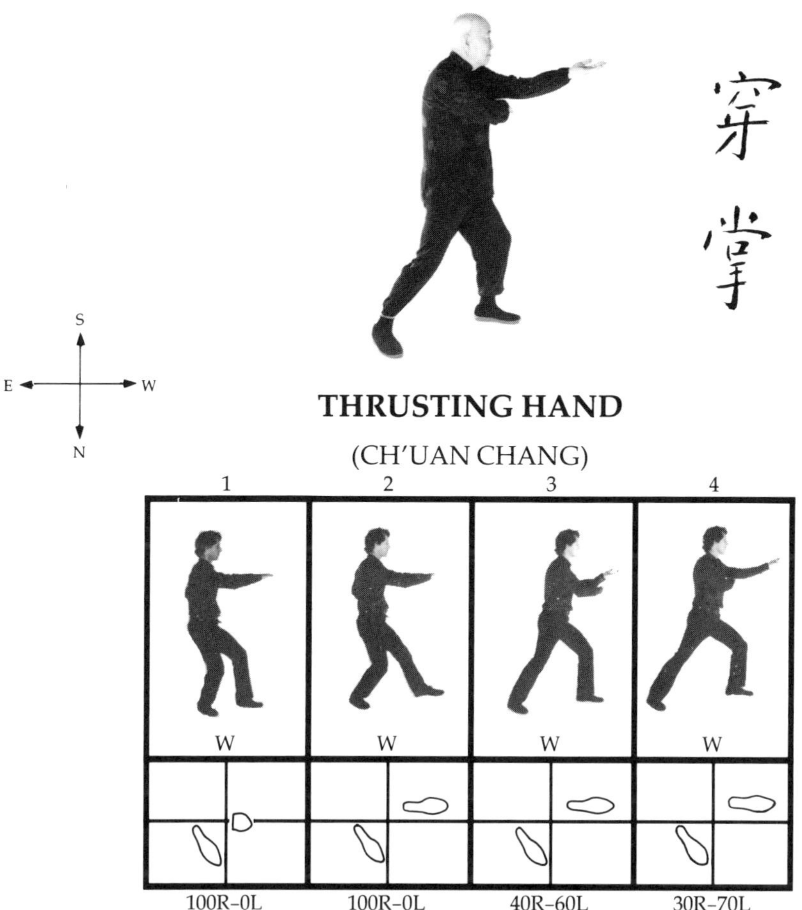

THRUSTING HAND

(CH'UAN CHANG)

During the Counts of:

1. Lower your body and bend your right knee slightly.
2. Take half a step with your left foot to the forward left direction with the heel touching first.
3. Withdraw your right hand. At the same time extend your left hand forward past the back of your hand. Gradually shift your weight to your left foot.
4. Shift 70% of your weight to the left foot. Continue to withdraw your right hand and to extend forward with your left hand until your right hand is under the left arm, near your left armpit, (with the palm down) and your left hand is in front at neck level with the palm upward and elbow slightly bent. You are still facing west.

POSTURE 134

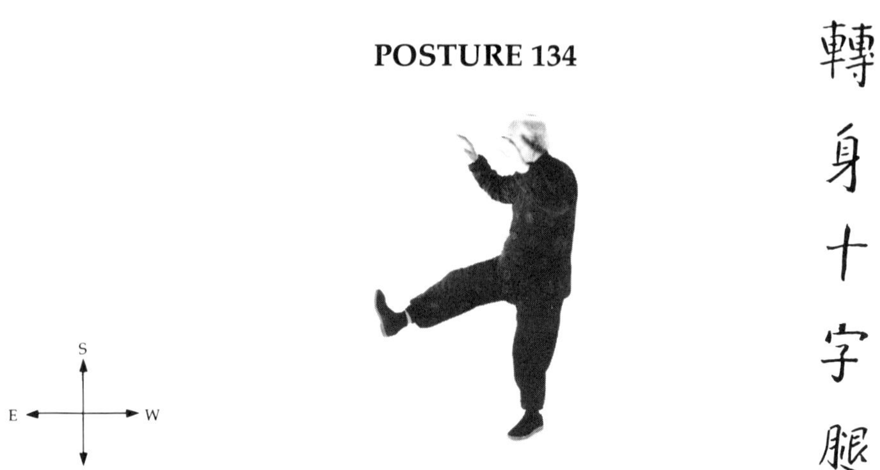

TURN AROUND AND KICK WITH SOLE (RIGHT FOOT)

(CHUAN SHEN TENG CHIO)

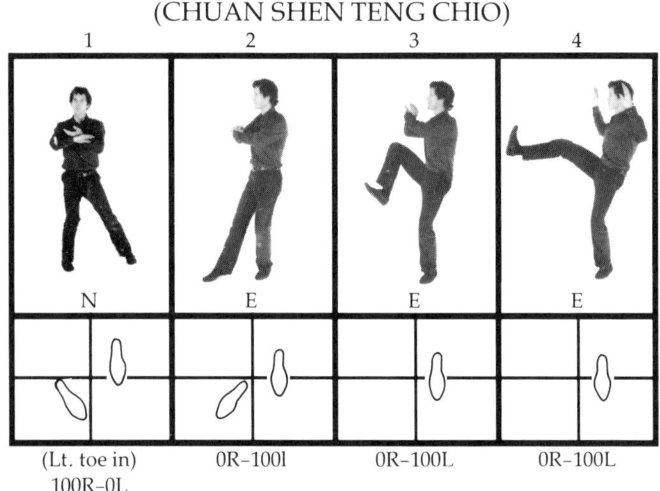

During the Counts of:

1. Bending the left arm and extending slightly the right arm, withdraw your left hand (palm up) on the back of your right hand (palm down) while you shift your weight to the right foot and gradually turn your body to the right (to face north). At the same time turn the left foot inward to point north.
2. Shift the weight to the left foot and let the right foot be brought onto the toes. At the same time circle the wrists so they remain close with the right hand on top, the left hand below and both palms downward. Turn your body to the right (east).
3. Turn the palms outward and at the same time raise your right leg with the knee bent and toes pointing diagonally upward.
4. Kick forward with your right sole with the toes upward while you extend the left hand outward to the north east corner and the right hand to the southeast corner. Both hands are nose level with the elbows well bent. Now you are facing east.

POSTURE 135

摟膝指襠捶

BRUSH KNEE AND PUNCH GROIN

(LOU HSI CHI TANG CH'UI)

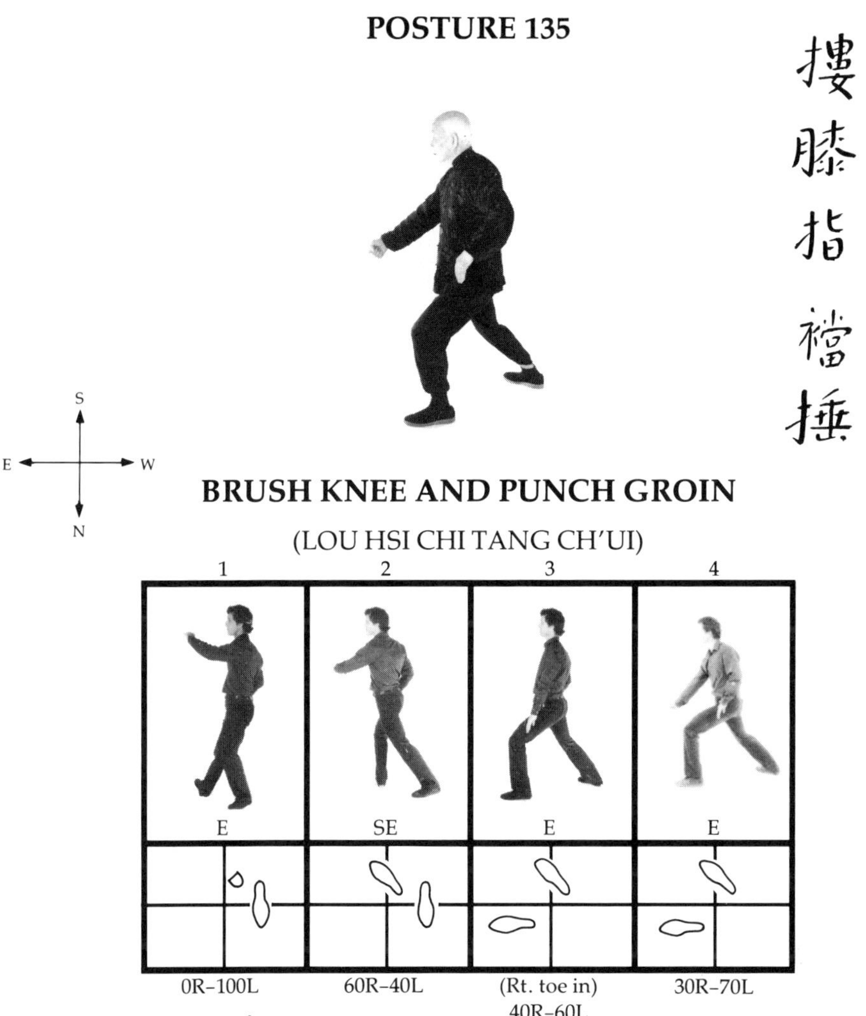

During the Counts of:

1. Lower and withdraw your left hand near the left side of your chest with the palm inward and lower your right leg with the foot touching (heel only) and toe pointing to the south. At the same time turn your body slightly to the right.
2. Continue to turn your body to the right (to face southeast). Shift your weight to the right leg. At the same time clench your right hand into a fist and place it at the right side of your waist with the "tiger-mouth" upward.
3. Take one big step forward with your left foot with the heel touching first and gradually shift your weight to it. Brush your left knee with your left palm and stop it beside the knee with the palm backward. Turn your right foot slightly inward.
4. Shift 70% of your weight to your left foot and strike out with your right fist toward your opponent's groin with the fist slightly downward and "tiger-mouth" upward. You are still facing east.

POSTURE 136

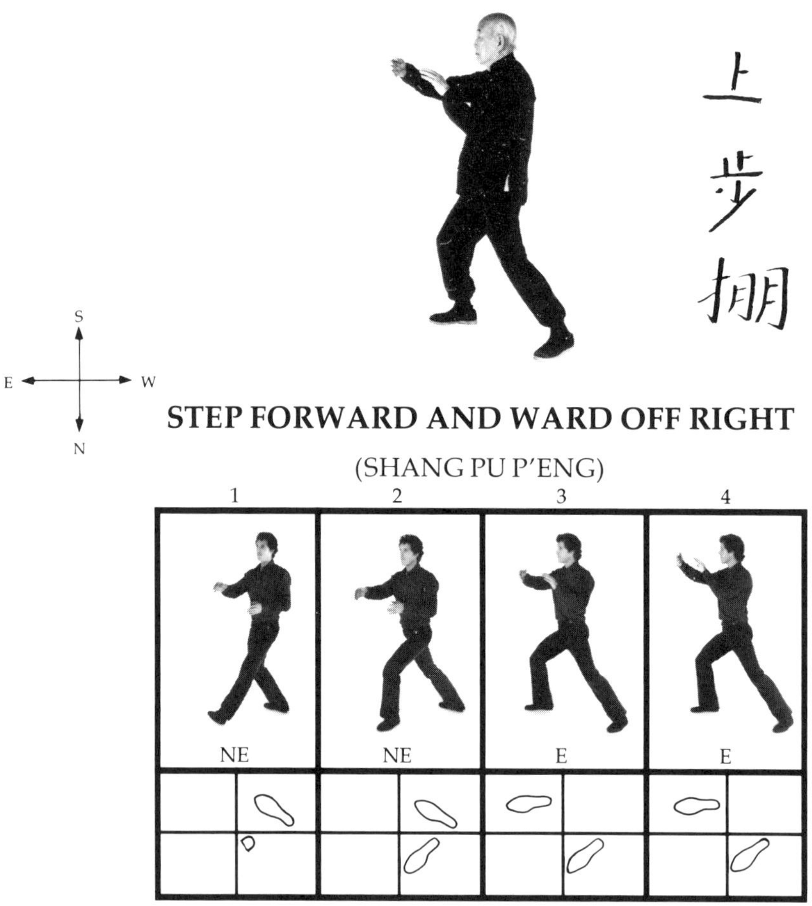

STEP FORWARD AND WARD OFF RIGHT

(SHANG PU P'ENG)

This posture is the same as posture #43.

POSTURE 137

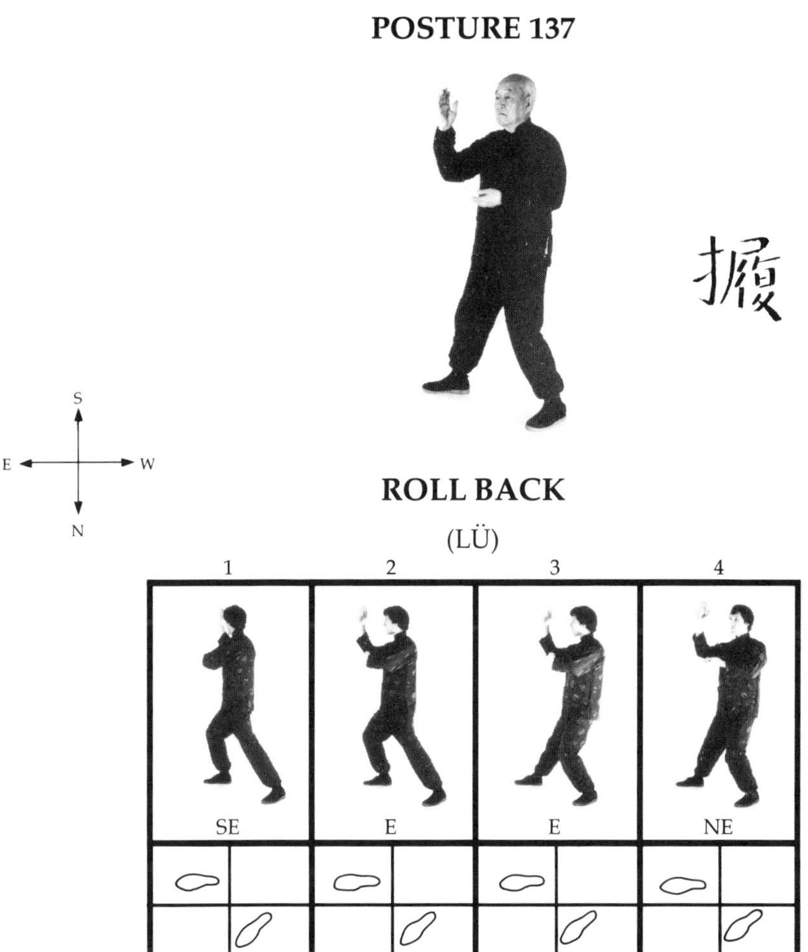

ROLL BACK

(LÜ)

This posture is the same as posture #5.

POSTURE 138

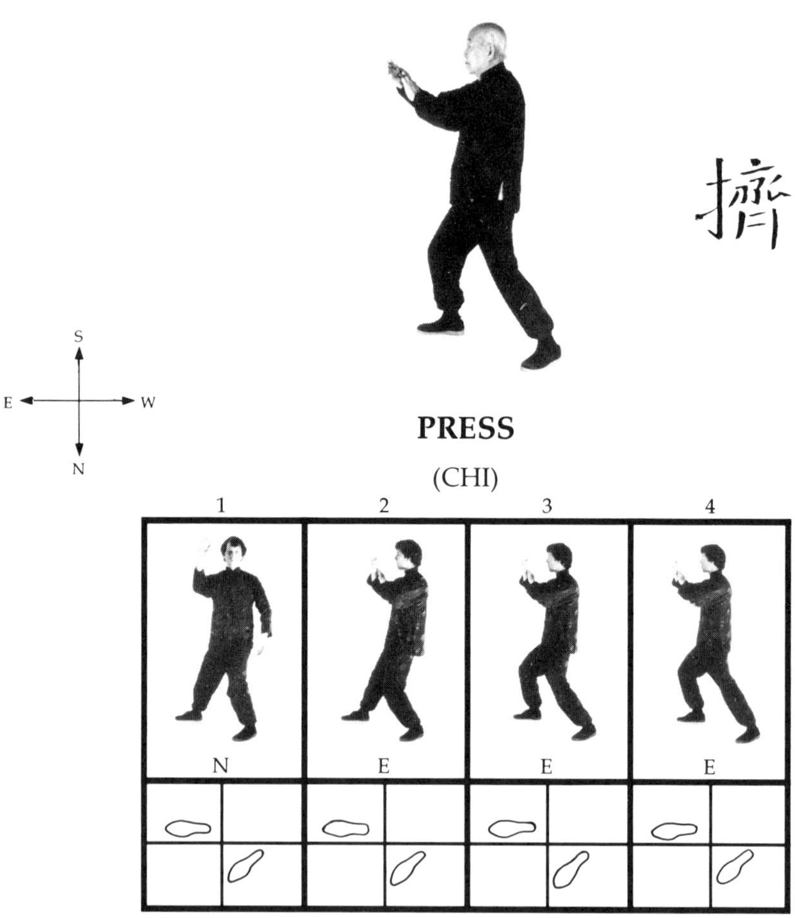

PRESS

(CHI)

This posture is the same as posture #6.

POSTURE 139

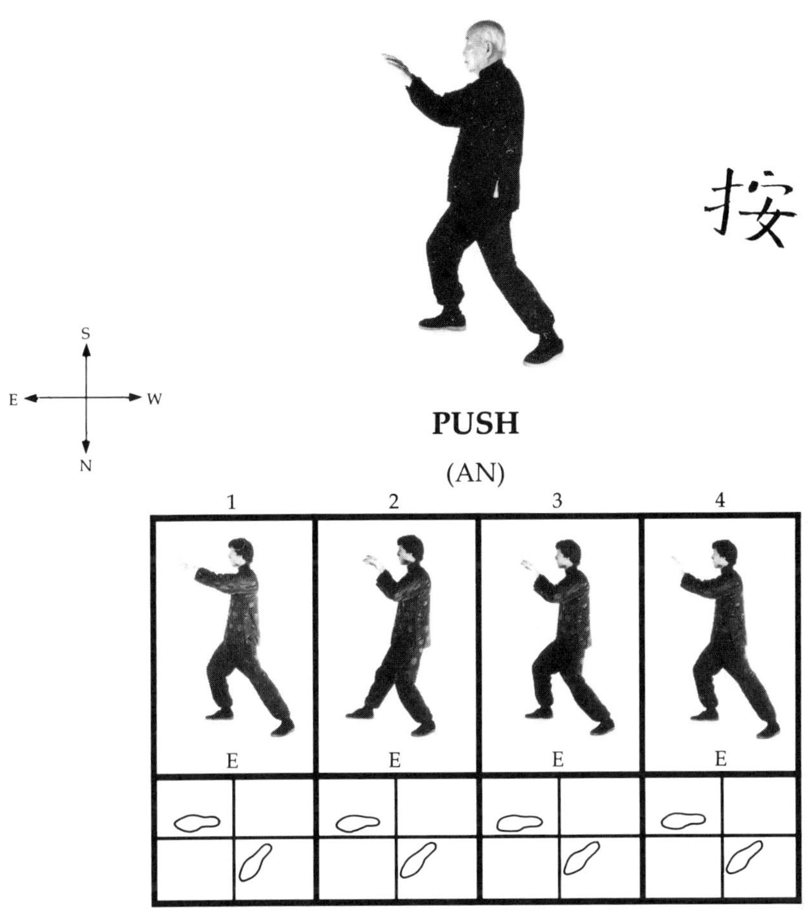

PUSH

(AN)

This posture is the same as posture #7.

POSTURE 140

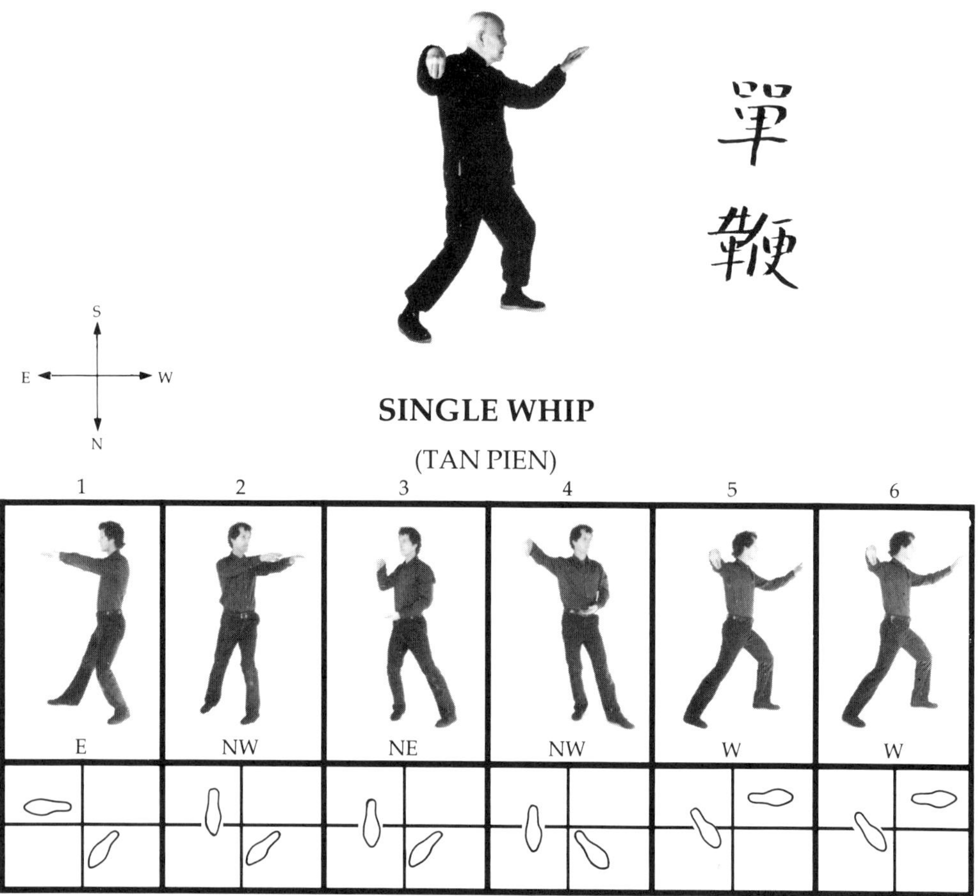

This posture is the same as posture #8.

POSTURE 141

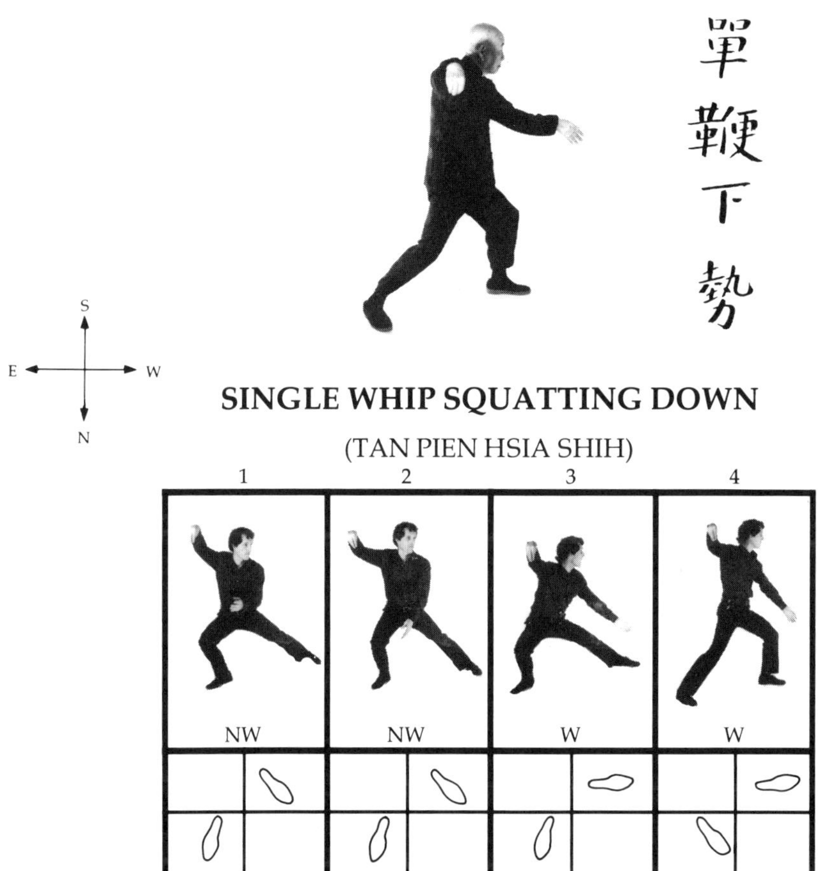

SINGLE WHIP SQUATTING DOWN

(TAN PIEN HSIA SHIH)

This posture is the same as posture #104.

POSTURE 142

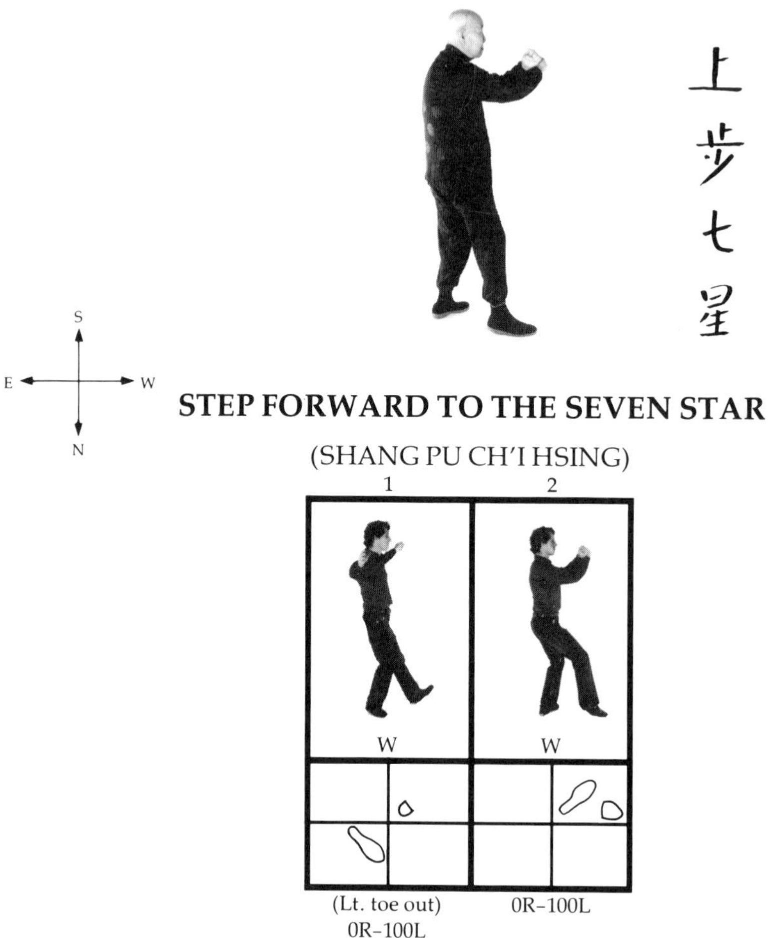

STEP FORWARD TO THE SEVEN STAR

(SHANG PU CH'I HSING)

During the Counts of:

1. Shift your entire weight to your right foot; toe out the left foot and then shift all the weight back onto the left foot. (Note: this picture does not show the beat at its completion; it shows the weight shift back and toe out only).
2. Take one-half step forward with your right foot with only the toes touching the ground, in front of the left foot. At the same time open your right "hook hand" and carry it in front of your chest, clenching both hands into fists. Join them at the wrists with the left hand inside of the right hand and "tiger-mouths" facing you. You are still facing west.

POSTURE 143

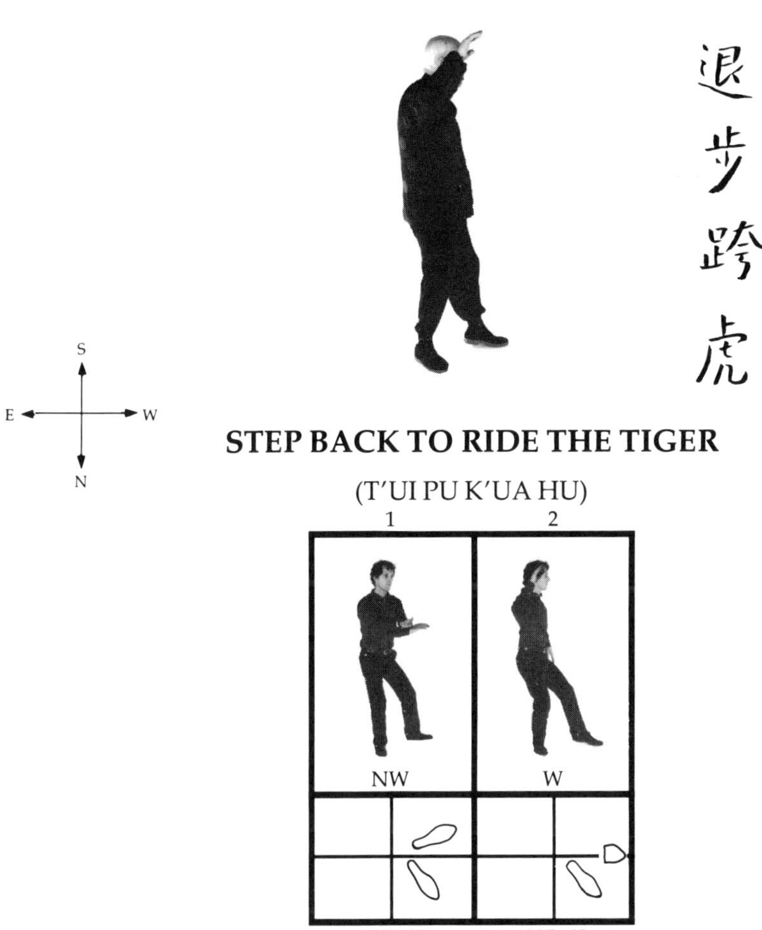

STEP BACK TO RIDE THE TIGER

(T'UI PU K'UA HU)

During the Counts of:

1. Draw back your right foot one step; set it down with the toes pointing northwest and shift the weight to it. At the same time turn your body slightly to the right, open your fists and circle both hands downward and backward.
2. Turn your body slightly to the left (to face west). Continue to circle your right hand backward and upward and hold it beside your right ear, with the fingers up, forearm vertical and palm forward. At the same time continue to lower your left hand and hold it beside your left hip joint with the palm backward. Shift your left foot slightly rightward, with only the toes touching the ground and the heel in line with your right heel. You are still facing west.

POSTURE 144

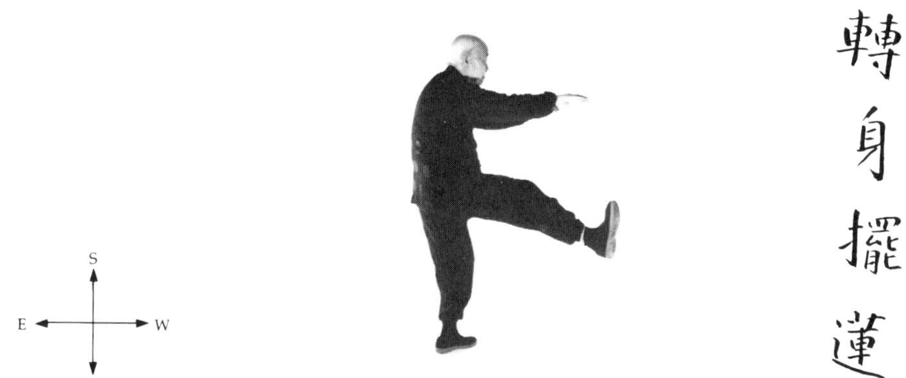

TURN AROUND AND SWEEP WITH LEG (RIGHT FOOT)

(CHUAN SHEN PAI LIEN)

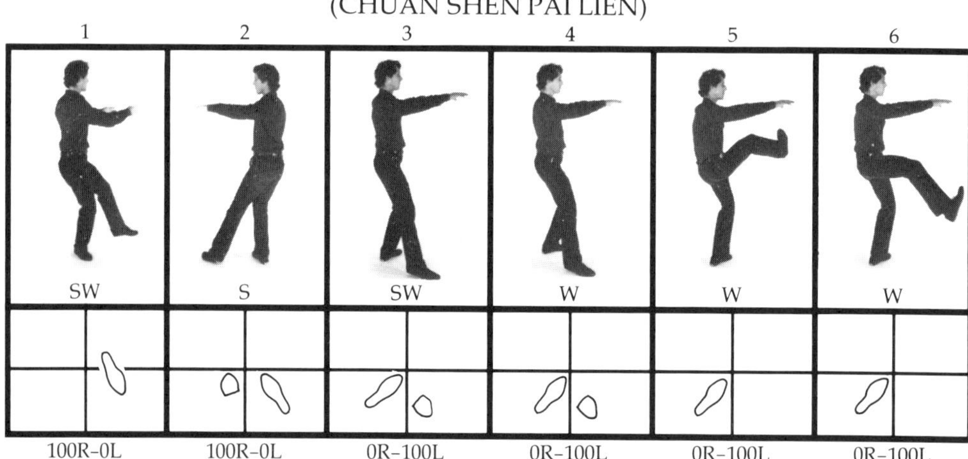

During the Counts of:

1. Turn your body slightly to the left (to face southwest), raise your left hand and lower your right hand extending them both to the southwest at chest height, so that they are parallel with the palms facing each other. At the same time shift your left foot slightly to the left with the toes pointing southwest and slightly off the ground.
2. Turn your palms downward and with the ball of your right foot on the ground, make a spinning turn to the right, (to face SE). Place your left foot down (on the toes) in front of your right foot with the left foot pointing southeast. The hands are parallel at shoulder height with the fingers pointing southeast.
3. Continue to turn your body to the right until you face west with the right toes facing northwest and hands parallel at shoulder height with the palms down. Gradually shift your weight to your left foot as the toes turn southwest.
4. Continue to turn your body to the right (NW) and shift your weight entirely to the left foot. At the same time pick up the right toes and circle your right foot slightly to the right and then place the toes on the ground pointing west.

5. Raise your right foot with the toes upward and circle the foot clockwise (leftward, upward and rightward) with the toes brushing your palms.
6. Continue to circle your right foot rightward at hip joint level with toes upward until the sole faces northwest. Now you are facing west.

POSTURE 145

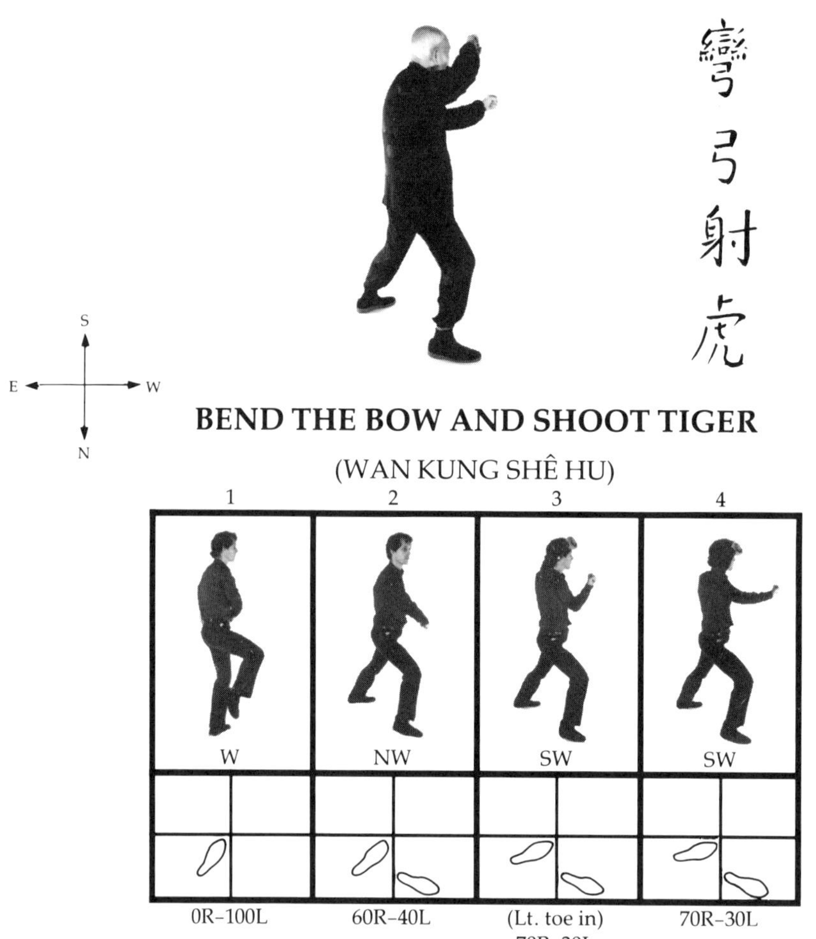

BEND THE BOW AND SHOOT TIGER

(WAN KUNG SHÊ HU)

During the Counts of:

1. Lower both hands near your left thigh with the palms facing each other. Lower your right leg near your left leg with the knee slightly bent, toes pointing down and foot slightly off the ground.
2. Step diagonally forward to the right (the heel touching first) with your right foot (northwest).
3. Gradually shift your weight to your right foot, turn your body to the left (to face southwest) and turn your left foot slightly inward. At the same time clench your hands into fists and circle them counterclockwise, rightward and upward so that your right fist is near your right ear with the knuckles inward and elbow bent, and your left fist is in front of your throat with the knuckles upward.
4. Extend your left fist forward to the southwest. The elbow is slightly bent with the "tiger-mouths" of both fists facing each other. You are now facing southwest.

POSTURE 146

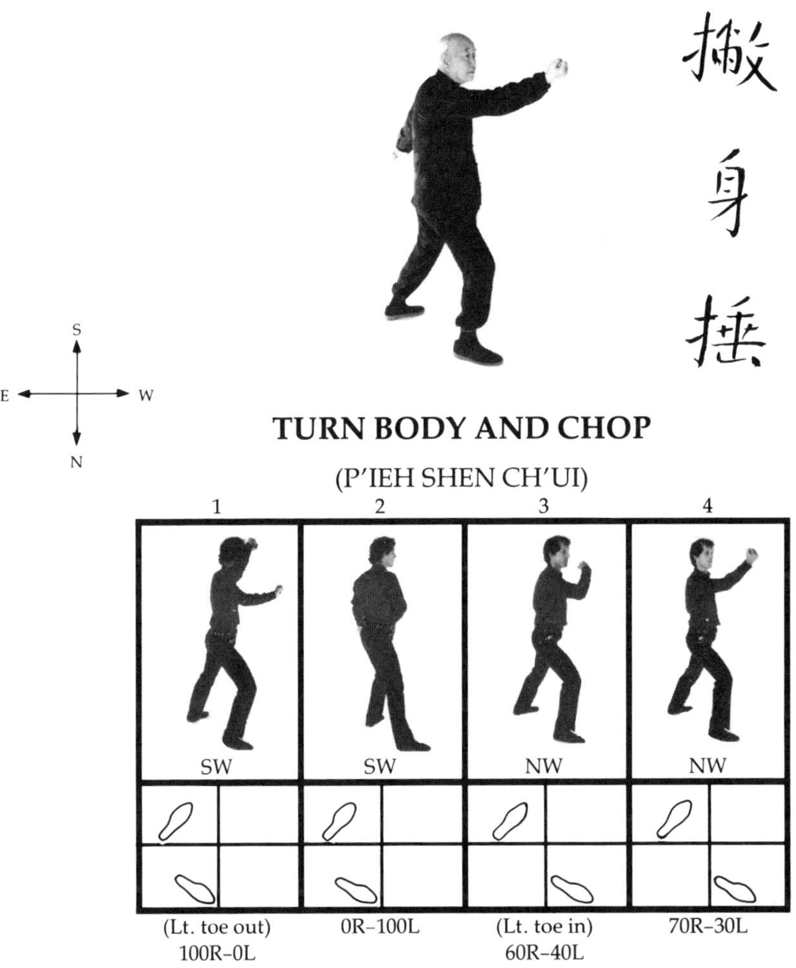

TURN BODY AND CHOP

(P'IEH SHEN CH'UI)

During the Counts of:

1. Raise your left foot off the ground and set it down with the foot turned slightly outward.
2. Shift your weight to the left foot, open your fists and lower both hands near your left thigh with the palms facing downward.
3. Take a short step diagonally to the right with your right foot (northwest) with the heel touching first, and shift your weight to it. Turn your left foot slightly inward. At the same time turn your body to the right (northwest) and clench your right hand into a fist.
4. Circle your right fist to the northwest in a diagonally upward direction with the knuckles downward. Extend your left hand backward at waist level with the palm down. You are now facing northwest.

POSTURE 147

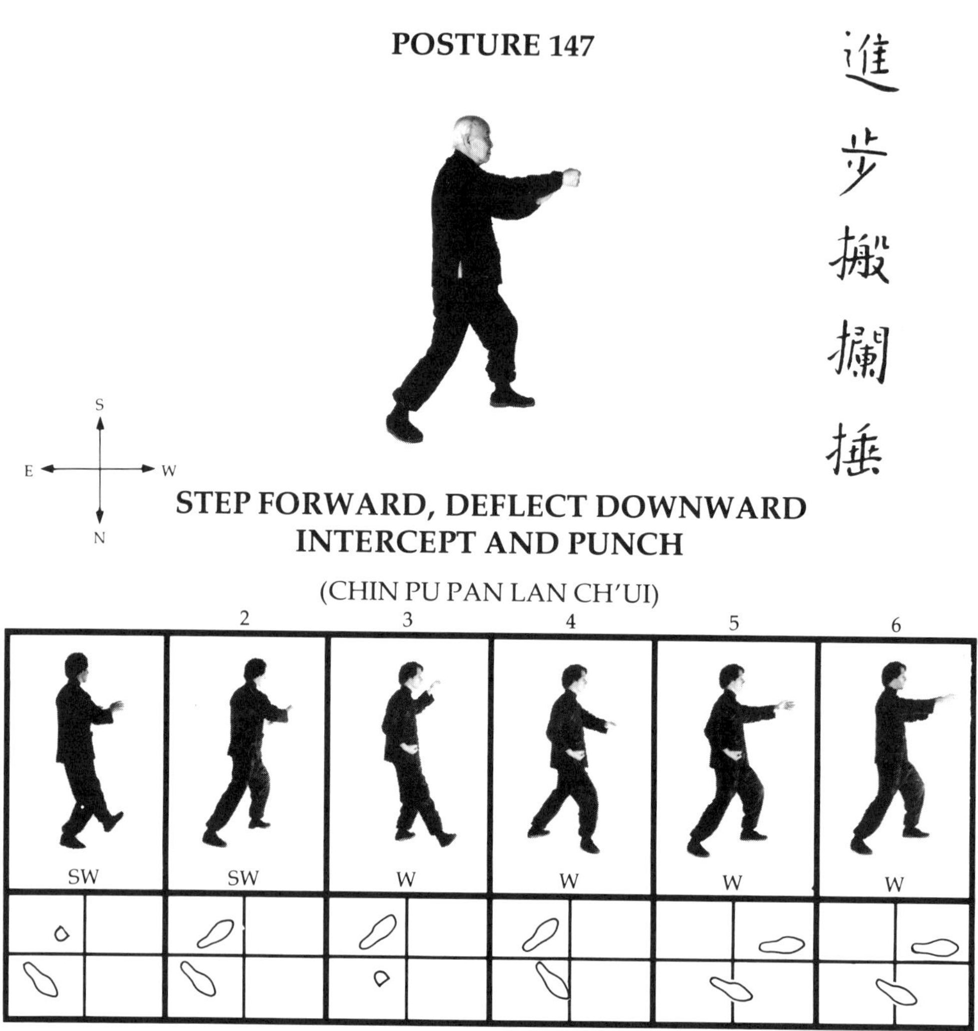

STEP FORWARD, DEFLECT DOWNWARD INTERCEPT AND PUNCH

(CHIN PU PAN LAN CH'UI)

During the Counts of:

1. Pick up your left foot and set it down with the foot turned slightly outward (SW).

Beats 2 to 6 are the same as the respective beats of posture #20.

POSTURE 148

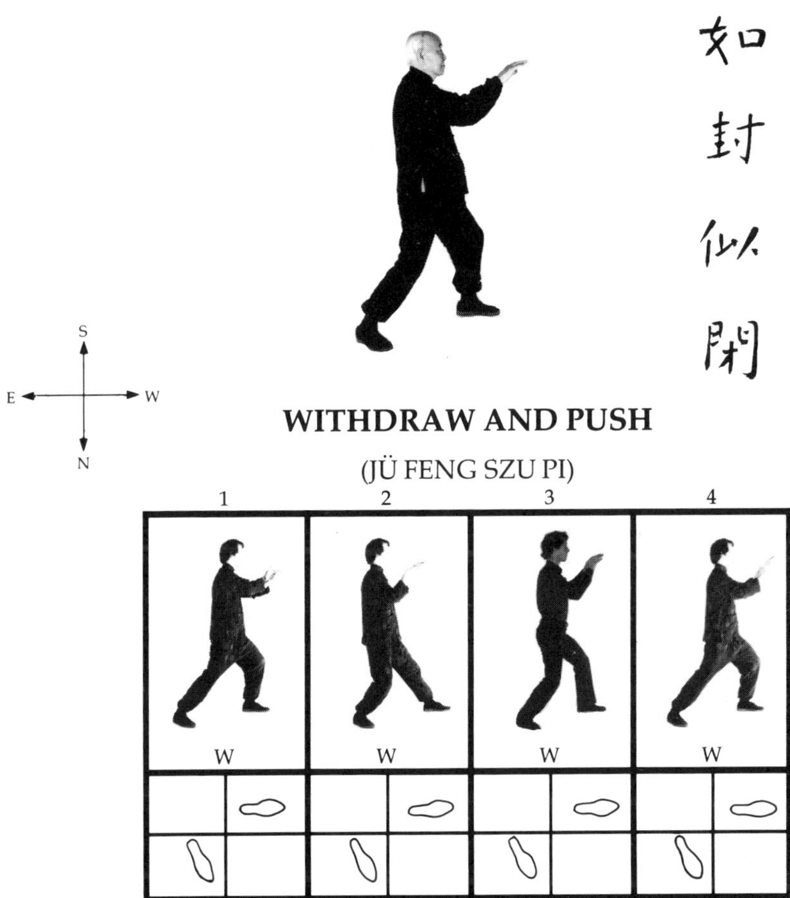

WITHDRAW AND PUSH

(JÜ FENG SZU PI)

This posture is the same as posture #21.

POSTURE 149

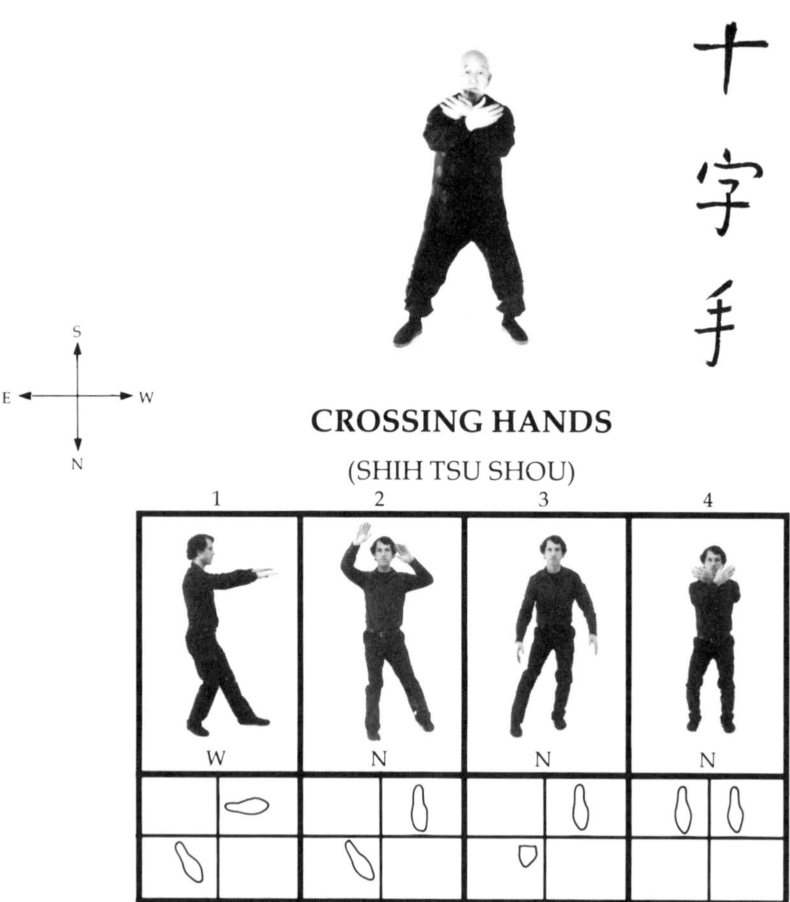

CROSSING HANDS

(SHIH TSU SHOU)

This posture is the same as posture #22.

POSTURE 150

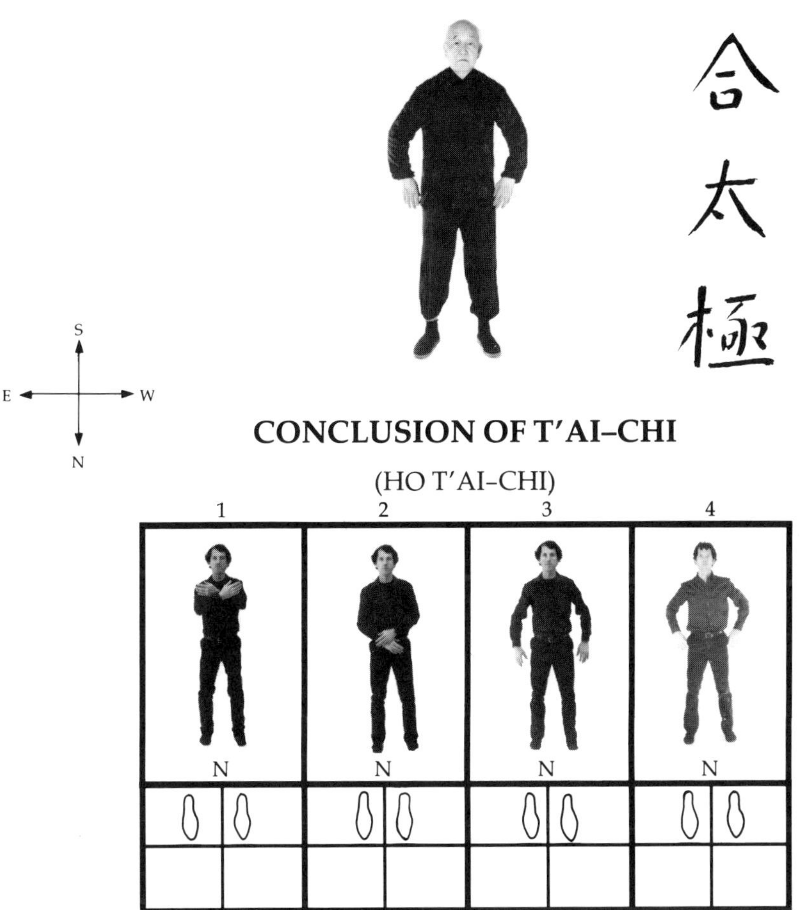

CONCLUSION OF T'AI-CHI

(HO T'AI-CHI)

During the Counts of:

1. Gradually raise your body and begin to lower your hands with the palms down. Shift the weight equally to both legs.
2. Continue to raise your body and lower your hands near your waist.
3. Separate your hands and bring them beside the thighs, with the fingers down.
4. Bend your elbows slightly with the palms backward. The center of gravity is between the two feet. You are now facing north.

T'ai Chi Ch'uan

Posture Reference Guide

Yang Style School
Master T. T. Liang

Body Direction Upon Completion	Rhythm	
N.	2	1. Preparation
N.	6	2. Beginning
N.	6	3. Ward Off, Left
E.	4	4. Ward Off, Right
NE.	4	5. Roll Back
E.	4	6. Press
E.	4	7. Push
W.	6	8. Single Whip
N.	2	9. Lifting Hands
N.	2	10. Shoulder Stroke
W.	2	11. White Crane Spreading Wings
W.	4	12. Brush Left Knee and Twist Step
W.	2	13. Playing The Guitar
W.	4	14. Brush Left Knee and Twist Step
W.	4	15. Brush Right Knee and Twist Step
W.	4	16. Brush Left Knee and Twist Step
W.	2	17. Playing the Guitar
W.	4	18. Brush Left Knee and Twist Step
NW.	2	19. Chop with Fist
W.	6	20. Step Forward, Deflect Downward, Intercept and Punch
W.	4	21. Withdraw and Push
N.	4	22. Crossing Hands
SE.	4	23. Embrace the Tiger and Return to the Mountain
E.	4	24. Roll Back
SE.	4	25. Press
SE.	4	26. Push
NW.	6	27. Slanging Single Whip
W.	6	28. Punch Under Elbow
W.	4	29. Step Back to Drive the Monkey Away (Right)
W.	4	30. Step Back to Drive the Monkey Away (Left)
W.	4	31. Step Back To Drive the Monkey Away (Right)
W.	4	32. Step Back to Drive the Monkey Away (Left)

W.	4	33. Step Back to Drive the Monkey Away (Right)
NE.	4	34. Diagonal Flying Posture
N.	2	35. Lifting Hands
N.	2	36. Shoulder Stroke
W.	2	37. White Crane Spreading Wings
W.	4	38. Brush Left Knee and Twist Step
W.	4	39. Needle At Sea Bottom
W.	4	40. Fan Penetrates the Back
E.	4	41. Turn Around and Chop
E.	6	42. Step Forward, Deflect Downward, Intercept and Punch
E.	4	43. Step Forward and Ward Off Right
NE.	4	44. Roll Back
E.	4	45. Press
E.	4	46. Push
W.	6	47. Single Whip
W.	4	48. Waving Hands in the Clouds (Left)
E.	4	49. Waving Hands in the Clouds (Right)
W.	4	50. Waving Hands in the Clouds (Left)
E.	4	51. Waving Hands in the Clouds (Right)
W.	4	52. Waving Hands in the Clouds (Left)
W.	4	53. Single Whip
W.	4	54. High Pat on Horse
NW.	6	55. Separating Right Foot
SW.	6	56. Separating Left Foot
E.	4	57. Turn Around and Strike with Heel (Left Foot)
E.	4	58. Brush Left Knee and Twist Step
E.	4	59. Brush Right Knee and Twist Step
E.	4	60. Step Forward and Punch Downward
W.	4	61. Turn Around and Chop with Fist
W.	6	62. Step Forward, Deflect Downward, Intercept and Punch
NW.	4	63. Kick Upward with Right Foot
SW.	4	64. Strike Tiger (Left Style)
NW.	4	65. Strike Tiger (Right Style)
NW.	4	66. Kick Upward with Right Foot
NW.	4	67. Strike with Both Fists
SW.	4	68. Kick Upward with Left Foot
W.	6	69. Turn Around and Kick with Sole (Right Foot)
NW.	2	70. Chop with Fist
W.	6	71. Step Forward, Deflect Downward, Intercept and Punch
W.	4	72. Withdraw and Push
N.	4	73. Crossing Hands
SE.	4	74. Embrace the Tiger and Return to the Mountain

E.	4	75. Roll Back
SE.	4	76. Press
SE.	4	77. Push
N.	6	78. Horizontal Single Whip
SE.	4	79. Parting Wild Horse's Mane, Right
NE.	4	80. Parting Wild Horse's Mane, Left
SE.	4	81. Parting Wild Horse's Mane, Right
N.	4	82. Ward Off, Left
E.	4	83. Ward Off, Right
NE.	4	84. Roll Back
E.	4	85. Press
E.	4	86. Push
W.	6	87. Single Whip
NE.	6	88. Fair Lady Weaving at Shuttle (1)
NW.	6	89. Fair Lady Weaving at Shuttle (2)
SW.	6	90. Fair Lady Weaving at Shuttle (3)
SE.	6	91. Fair Lady Weaving at Shuttle (4)
N.	4	92. Ward Off, Left
E.	4	93. Ward Off, Right
NE.	4	94. Roll Back
E.	4	95. Press
E.	4	96. Push
W.	6	97. Single Whip
W.	4	98. Waving Hands in the Clouds (Left)
E.	4	99. Waving Hands in the Clouds (Right)
W.	4	100. Waving Hands in the Clouds (Left)
E.	4	101. Waving Hands in the Clouds (Right)
W.	4	102. Waving Hands in the Clouds (Left)
W.	4	103. Single Whip
W.	4	104. Single Whip Squatting Down
W.	2	105. Golden Rooster Standing on One Leg (Right)
W.	2	106. Golden Rooster Standing on One Leg (Left)
W.	4	107. Step Back to Drive the Monkey Away (Right)
W.	4	108. Step Back to Drive the Monkey Away (Left)
W.	4	109. Step Back to Drive the Monkey Away (Right)
W.	4	110. Step Back to Drive the Monkey Away (Left)
W.	4	111. Step Back to Drive the Monkey Away (Right)
NE.	4	112. Diagonal Flying Posture
N.	2	113. Lifting Hands
N.	2	114. Shoulder Stroke
W.	2	115. White Crane Spreading Wings

W.	4	116. Brush Left Knee and Twist Step
W.	4	117. Needle at Sea Bottom
W.	4	118. Fan Penetrates the Back
E.	4	119. Turn Around and White Snake Puts out Tongue
E.	6	120. Step Forward, Deflect Downward, Intercept and Punch
E.	4	121. Step Forward and Ward Off Right
NE.	4	122. Roll Back
E.	4	123. Press
E.	4	124. Push
W.	6	125. Single Whip
W.	4	126. Waving Hands in the Clouds (Left)
E.	4	127. Waving Hands in the Clouds (Right)
W.	4	128. Waving Hands in the Clouds (Left)
E.	4	129. Waving Hands in the Clouds (Right)
W.	4	130. Waving Hands in the Clouds (Left)
W.	4	131. Single Whip
W.	4	132. High Pat on Horse
W.	4	133. Thrusting Hand
E.	4	134. Turn Around and Kick with Sole (Right Foot)
E.	4	135. Brush Knee and Punch Groin
E.	4	136. Step Forward and Ward Off Right
NE.	4	137. Roll Back
E.	4	138. Press
E.	4	139. Push
W.	6	140. Single Whip
W.	4	141. Single Whip Squatting Down
W.	2	142. Step Forward to the Seven Stars
W.	2	143. Step Back to Ride the Tiger
W.	6	144. Turn Around and Sweep with Leg (Right Foot)
SW.	4	145. Bend the Bow and Shoot Tiger
NW.	4	146. Turn Body and Chop
W.	6	147. Step Forward, Deflect Downward, Intercept and Punch
W.	4	148. Withdraw and Push
N.	4	149. Crossing Hands
N.	4	150. Conclusion of T'ai-Chi

The Ten Guiding Points of T'ai–Chi Ch'uan

(T'ai–Chi Ch'uan Chih yao)

1) To relax. (Sung)
2) To sink. (Chen)
3) To concentrate your line of vision. (Yen shen chu shih)
4) The chest should be held in, the back straightened, the shoulders and elbows lowered. (Han Hsuing pa pei, chen chien chui chow)
5) The head should be upright and the lowest vertebrae plumb erect. (Hsi ling ting ching, wei lu chung cheng)
6) The substantial and the insubstantial must be clearly discriminated. (Hsu shih ui fen Ching chu)
7) All the movements are to be directed by the mind instead of by external muscular force. (Yung yi pu yung li)
8) Meditation in action, action in meditation. (Tung Chung Ghui ching; Ching Ghung chiu tung)
9) Up and down follow immediately; the whole body acts as one unit. (Shand hsia Hsiang hsui: Ghuan shen yi chih)
10) All the movements are to be connected without severance. (Hsiang lien pu tuan)

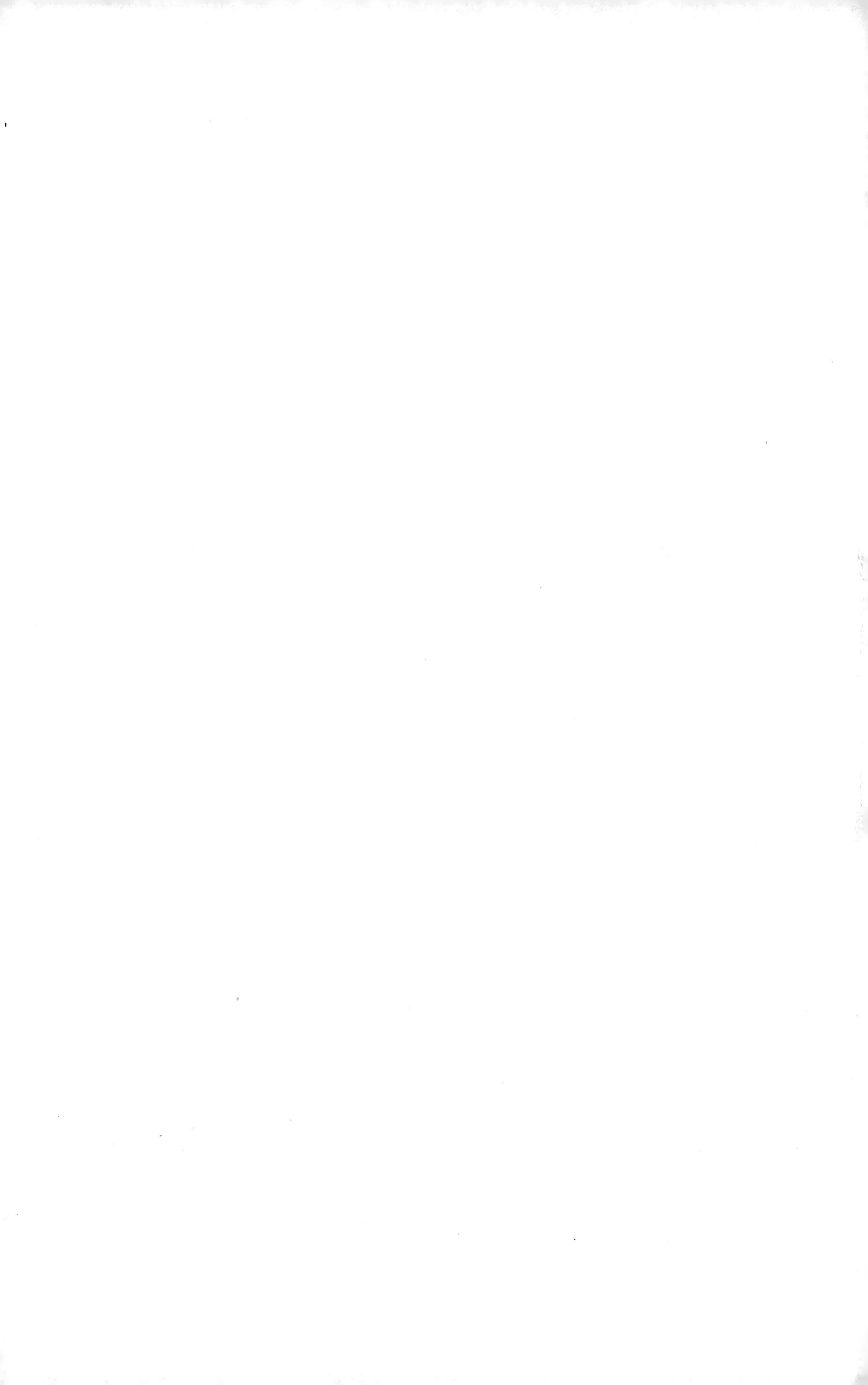

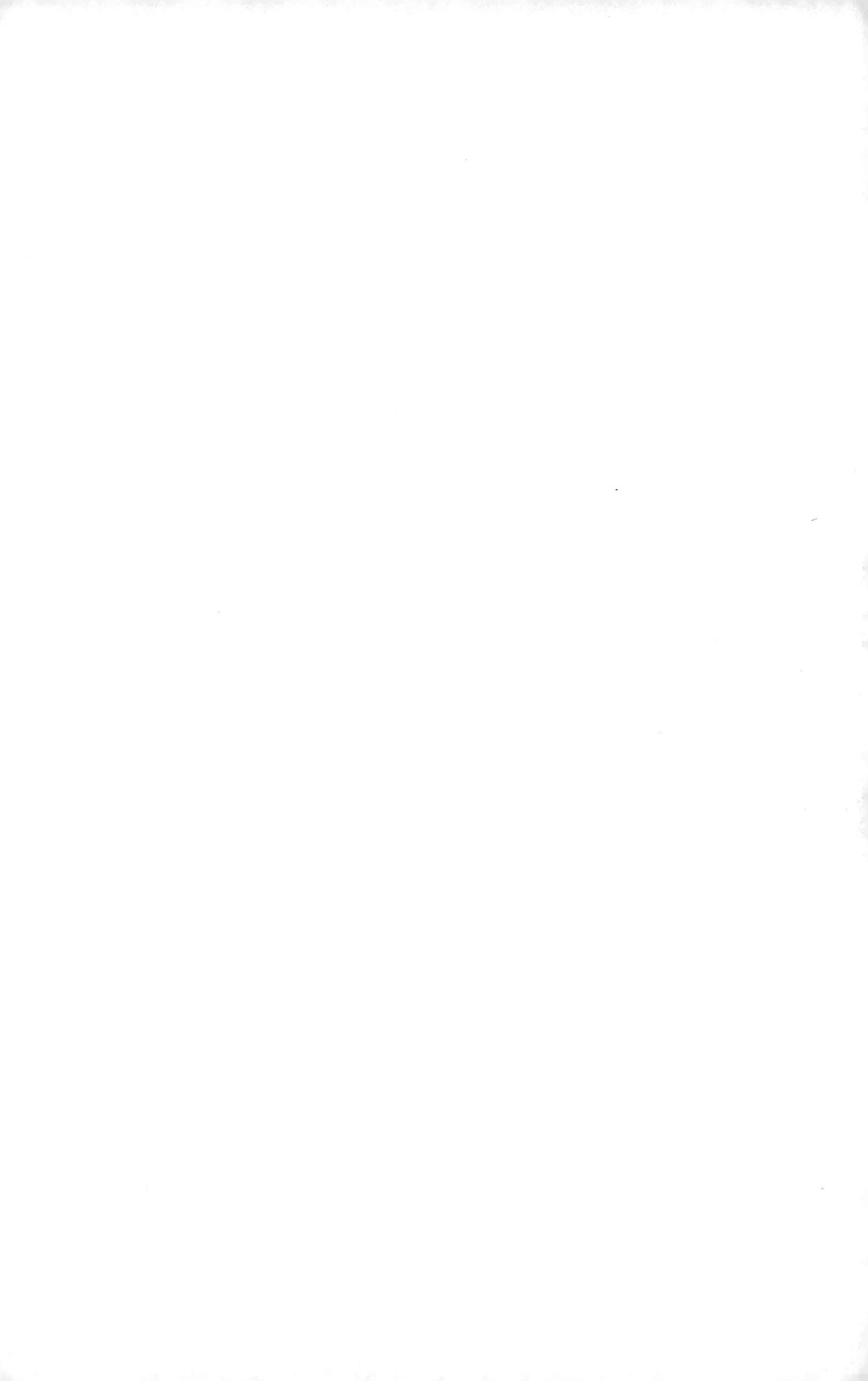

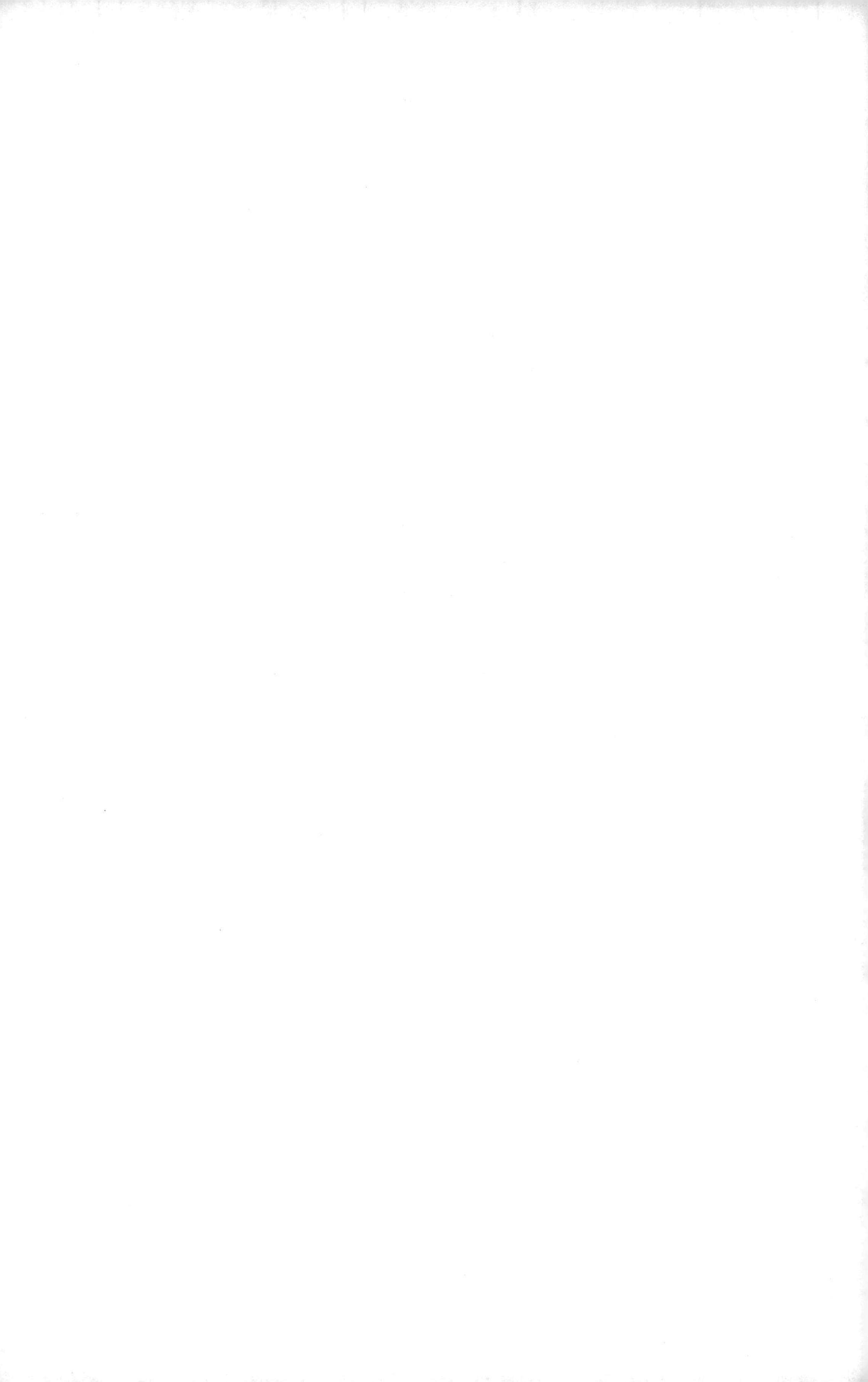

PRINTED IN CANADA